Obesity
Care and
Bariatric Surgery

Obesity
Care and
Bariatric Surgery

Editors

Kenric M Murayama
University of Hawaii, USA

Shanu N Kothari
Gundersen Lutheran Health System, USA

W⦾ World Scientific

NEW JERSEY · LONDON · SINGAPORE · BEIJING · SHANGHAI · HONG KONG · TAIPEI · CHENNAI · TOKYO

Published by

World Scientific Publishing Co. Pte. Ltd.

5 Toh Tuck Link, Singapore 596224

USA office: 27 Warren Street, Suite 401-402, Hackensack, NJ 07601

UK office: 57 Shelton Street, Covent Garden, London WC2H 9HE

Library of Congress Cataloging-in-Publication Data
Obesity care and bariatric surgery / [edited by] Kenric M. Murayama, Shanu N. Kothari.
    p. ; cm.
  Includes bibliographical references.
  ISBN 978-9814699303 (hardcover : alk. paper)
  I. Murayama, Kenric M., editor. II. Kothari, Shanu N., editor.
  [DNLM: 1. Bariatric Surgery--methods. 2. Obesity, Morbid--surgery.
3. Treatment Outcome. WI 900]
  RD540.5
  617.4'3--dc23

                           2015026561

British Library Cataloguing-in-Publication Data
A catalogue record for this book is available from the British Library.

Typeset by Stallion Press
Email: enquiries@stallionpress.com

Contents

Preface   vii

Chapter 1.   Obesity-Related Health Issues   1
             Rajasree Nambron and Daniel K. Short

Chapter 2.   History of Bariatric Surgery   11
             Joshua D. Pfeiffer and Shanu N. Kothari

Chapter 3.   Roux-en-Y Gastric Bypass: Indications,
             Procedures and Outcomes   29
             Umer I. Chaudhry and Dean J. Mikami

Chapter 4.   Biliopancreatic Diversion and Duodenal
             Switch: Indications, Procedure and Outcomes   37
             Patrick Fei and Fernando Bonanni

Chapter 5.   Sleeve Gastrectomy: Indications, Procedure
             and Outcomes   55
             Yalini Vigneswaran and Michael B. Ujiki

Chapter 6.   Comparative Outcomes in Bariatric Surgery   67
             Christopher R. Daigle and Stacy A. Brethauer

Chapter 7. Complications of Bariatric Surgery and
            Management   77
            Bill Ran Luo and Alex Nagle

Chapter 8. Innovations in Bariatric Surgery   97
            *George Pontikis, Pornthep Prathanvanich
            and Bipan Chand*

Chapter 9. Nutrition After Bariatric Surgery   113
            Karen Buzby and Danielle Rosenfeld Staub

Chapter 10. Metabolic Impact of Bariatric Surgery   147
            Aileen A. Murphy and Kevin M. Reavis

Index   161

Preface

Kenric M. Murayama, MD

Obesity is a major public health issue and has moved from a disease on the periphery to one that is approaching epidemic proportions. The burden of obesity on our healthcare system is difficult to accurately estimate, but the economic impact resulting from the medical and psychosocial issues is burgeoning. One important result of the increased interest and attention obesity is receiving is the development of new treatment options and research endeavors.

In this text, the expert group of authors has presented comprehensive reviews of a number of critical discussion points related to obesity including a discussion of the obesity-related health issues, a history of bariatric surgery, nutrition issues after bariatric surgery, and the metabolic impact of bariatric surgery. The text is intended to provide the reader with both a comprehensive overview of the management of obesity and quick reviews of specific topics in obesity care.

Chapter 1

Obesity-Related Health Issues

Rajasree Nambron[*] and Daniel K. Short[†,‡,§]

*Department of Internal Medicine, Gundersen Health System,
1836 South Avenue, La Crosse, WI 54601, USA
†Department of Endocrinology, Gundersen Health System,
1836 South Avenue, La Crosse, WI 54601, USA
‡dkshort@gundersenhealth.org

The prevalence of both overweight and obesity are increasing in the United States and worldwide. More than one third of adults in the US are currently obese.[1] The estimated financial impact of obesity in 2008 was over 140 billion dollars,[2] including both direct and indirect costs. The health impact of obesity, including morbidity and mortality, is devastating. Both years of life and quality of life are affected; obesity at age 40 decreases life expectancy by 7 years,[3] and the quality-adjusted years of life lost in the USA due to obesity and obesity related diseases have doubled recently.[4] It is estimated that obesity leads to between 111,000 and 365,000 excess deaths annually in the United States. WHO describes obesity as most visible but neglected health issue affecting both developed and developing countries.[5]

The accepted definition of overweight is a body mass index (BMI) of 25 kg/m^2 or above, and obesity is defined as a BMI of 30 kg/m^2 and above.

---

§Corresponding author.

Table 1 Classification of overweight and obesity by BMI.

	Obesity Class	BMI (kg/m^2)
Underweight	—	<18.5
Normal	—	18.5–24.9
Overweight	—	25–29.9
Obesity	Class I	30–34.9
	Class II	35–39.9
Severe Obesity	Class III	>40

Economic impact: It has recently been estimated that the financial cost of obesity is approximately 190 billion dollars annually in the US.[4,6] A study from the Mayo Clinic reported that obese employees accumulate 1,850 dollars more in medical costs than their healthy counterparts each year. For an employee with BMI of 35–40, the cost was actually 3,000 dollars annually.[6] It is estimated that it costs 5 billion dollars annually for the extra jet fuel needed to fly heavier Americans. The cost of excess absenteeism for male and female workers with BMI > 40 is estimated to be over 1,000 dollars per year.[6]

Health Risks

Obesity is strongly associated with the development of premature cardiovascular disease. There are several other major physical and mental conditions associated with obesity. These are briefly outlined in the following sections.

Hypertension:

Data from NHANES III show that as BMI increases, blood pressures increases proportionally.[7] For example, a person with 10 kg higher body weight will have on average 2 mm Hg higher systolic and 2.3 mm Hg higher diastolic pressures, according to the results of a large international study (INTERSALT), involving over 10,000 men and women.[8]

Dyslipidemia:

The pattern of dyslipidemia seen with obesity includes high triglycerides, high total cholesterol and low high density lipoproteins (HDL) combined with normal or high low density lipoproteins (LDL). Several studies have shown that as BMI increases there is an increase in triglyceride levels.[9] This is true in both men and women and at all ages. Weight gain, overweight and obesity have all been shown to increase cholesterol levels. People with a higher waist circumference have also been shown to have a higher total cholesterol.

Diabetes Mellitus:

Several studies including the Nurse's Health Study have shown that there is an increased relative risk of developing diabetes with an increase in BMI over 25 kg/m^2.[10] It has also been shown that abdominal obesity is an independent risk factor for developing diabetes.

Coronary artery disease:

Increases in weight lead to higher levels of total cholesterol, LDL cholesterol and triglycerides, as noted above. Also fibrinogen increases, insulin resistance may develop and blood pressure may rise as well. These changes in turn can lead to adverse coronary outcomes. CHD risk is lowest in men and women with BMI lower than 22 and then rises progressively with increases in BMI.[11] For example, a gain of 5–8 kg in weight leads to a 25% increase in myocardial infarction incidence and CHD related deaths. This has been shown in several populations around the world.[11] The co-morbid conditions associated with obesity, such as diabetes, hypertension and hyperlipidemia likely contribute to the increased vascular risk.

Atrial flutter/fibrillation:

In an analysis of over 5,000 patients in the Framingham study, patients with a BMI > 30 kg/m2 were prone to have atrial fibrillation.[12] Other studies have shown an increase in both atrial flutter and atrial fibrillation in obese patients without any underlying cardiac disease.[13]

Congestive heart failure (CHF):

CHF is a complication of obesity which has been identified in several studies, and is a major cause of death.[14] With increasing weight gain, the heart muscle is affected, with a resulting increase in left ventricular mass. Obesity leads to an increased blood volume and high cardiac output which causes eccentric hypertrophy and diastolic dysfunction. This is worse in the setting of coexisting diabetes and hypertension. Excess wall stress can ultimately lead to systolic dysfunction as well. Obesity hypoventilation syndrome and hypoxemia and obstructive sleep apnea cause hypoxemia and can also lead to congestive heart failure.

Stroke:

An increased risk of ischemic stroke has been reported with increasing BMI. As an example, the Nurse's Health Study reported an increased risk of ischemic stroke in women whose BMI was over 27 kg/m2.[15] An increased risk of both hemorrhagic and ischemic stroke has been reported in men as well.[15,16] In a study with over 85,000 participants, an increased risk of stoke was seen with every standard deviation of increase in BMI, waist circumference and waist to hip ratio.[17]

Sleep apnea:

Sleep apnea is strongly associated with obesity and diabetes. Sleep apnea can lead to pulmonary hypertension and right heart strain. Due to increased abdominal pressure, obese patients exhibit increased residual volume, decreased lung compliance and reduced respiratory drive. Obstructive sleep apnea and obesity hypoventilation syndrome cause significant morbidity and also generate considerable costs to the medical system in terms of both medical care and hospitalizations.

GERD:

Obesity is a strong risk factor for gastroesophaegeal reflux disease and esophagitis, likely due to increased intra-abdominal pressure. GERD may improve with weight loss.

Hepato-biliary disease:

Both Nurse's Health Study and Health Professionals Study have noted an increased incidence of symptomatic gallstone disease in patients with increasing BMI.[18] There is increased likelihood of precipitation of cholesterol within the gallbladder with increases in the biliary concentration of cholesterol with respect to bile acids, such as occurs with obesity. Steatosis is seen on liver biopsy in patients with obesity, mainly due to increased synthesis of triglycerides in excess of clearance, leading to accumulation in liver.[18]

Cancer:

Increasing BMI in both men and women is associated with increased mortality from cancer of esophagus, colon, rectum, liver, gall bladder and pancreas. The incidence of renal cancer, non-Hodgkin lymphoma, multiple myeloma and cancers of the reproductive system in both men and women are also increased in the obese population.[19]

Deep venous thrombosis (DVT):

There is an increase incidence of DVT and pulmonary embolism seen with increasing BMI. There is actually a decrease in risk in underweight individuals as well.[20] The risk of recurrent DVT is also increased in the obese. Some of the increase in thrombosis risk may be due to the decrease in activity that is seen in the obese population. Obese patients also have a significantly increased risk of chronic venous stasis changes in the lower extremities.

Endocrine changes:

As noted previously, diabetes and dyslipidemia are the dominant endocrine problems related to obesity. Other endocrine problems include decreased fertility in women, which is associated with both an ovulatory cycles and irregular menses that are seen with obesity, and leads to an increased utilization of assisted reproductive technology in this population. There is also an increased risk of pregnancy-induced hypertension and cesarean delivery in obese women. In men, obesity is an independent risk factor for erectile dysfunction.[21]

Genitourinary disease:

Several published studies report that obesity is an independent risk factor for developing chronic kidney disease (Framingham Offspring study, Hypertension Detection and Follow-up program and Multiphasic Health testing Service program).[22] Other specific kidney disorders include focal segmental glomerular-sclerosis, reversible obesity-related glomerulopathy and kidney stones. In women, obesity is a risk for urinary incontinence.

Pseudotumor cerebri (Idiopathic Intracranial Hypertension):

Pseudo tumor cerebri is a syndrome that includes symptoms of hypertension, visual loss and papilledema, normal CSF constitution elevated opening pressure on lumbar puncture and normal neuroimaging. Obesity is a major risk factor for this syndrome, especially in childbearing women. In men this risk may be less prevalent. The annual incidence may be as high as 1 to 2 per 100,000 per year.[23]

Osteoarthritis:

Obesity significantly contributes to the onset of osteoarthritis, especially of knees and ankles. Excess weight causes wear and tear to the cartilage and also alters the cartilage and bone metabolism independent of weight bearing.[24] One study in women showed that a decrease in BMI decreased the odds of developing osteoarthritis by over 50%.[25]

Skin changes:

The most common skin changes are stretch marks (striae) due to fat deposits expanding the subcutaneous tissue. Acanthosis nigricans around neck, axillae and knuckles due to hyperinsulinemia (insulin resistance) is another feature of obesity. Hirsutism in women due to increased testosterone is seen especially with visceral obesity.

Psychosocial dysfunction:

There is a stigma seen in education, employment and health that has been shown in several studies.[26] In a report where over 10,000 adolescents were looked at, women with BMI over the 95th percentile of age and sex, completed fewer years of school , were 20% less likely to be married, and had lower household incomes compared to normal subjects. Men who were overweight were 11% less likely to be married than their normal weight counterparts. Obesity also leads to an increased risk of depression, especially in younger women.

Conclusion

Obesity is a common health problem with significant associated morbidity and mortality. It causes dysfunction in multiple organ systems, and can lead to significant psychosocial morbidity as well. Improved recognition of obesity as a serious health issue by the medical community is urgently needed, as are improved treatments for this condition. Only by directly addressing the problem of obesity, the obesity-related complications such as diabetes and cardiovascular disease be adequately addressed and prevented.

References

1. Ogden CL, Carroll MD, Kit BK, Flegal KM. (2012) Prevalence of obesity in the United States, 2009–2010. NCHS Data Brief (82): 1–8.
2. Finkelstein, EA, Trogdon, JG, Cohen, JW, and Dietz, W. (2009) Annual medical spending attributable to obesity: Payer- and service-specific estimates. *Health Affairs* **28**(5): w822–w831.
3. Jia H, Lubetkin EI. (2010) Obesity-related quality-adjusted life years lost in the U.S. from 1993 to 2008. *Am J Prev Med* **39**(3): 220–7.
4. Peeters A, Barendregt JJ, Willekens F, Mackenbach JP, Al Mamun A, Bonneux L. (2003) NEDCOM, the Netherlands Epidemiology and Demography Compression of Morbidity Research Group. Obesity in adulthood and its consequences for life expectancy: A life-table analysis. *Ann Intern Med* **138**(1): 24–32.

5. WHO. (2000) *Obesity: Preventing and managing the global epidemic.* WHO Technical Report Series number 894. Geneva: WHO.
6. Moriarty JP, Branda ME, Olsen KD, Shah ND, Borah BJ, Wagie AE, Egginton JS, Naessens JM. (2012) The effects of incremental costs of smoking and obesity on health care costs among adults: a 7-year longitudinal study. *J Occup Environ Med* **54**(3): 286–91.
7. CDC. (2009) *National Health and Nutrition Examination Survey (NHANES): Health tech/blood pressure procedures manual.* Hyattsville, MD, US Department of Health and Human Services, CDC, National Center for Health Statistics; Available at http://www.cdc.gov/nchs/data/nhanes/nhanes_09_10/BP.pdf.
8. Dyer AR, Elliott P. (1989) The INTERSALT study: Relations of body mass index to blood pressure. INTERSALT Co-operative Research Group. *J Hum Hypertens* **3**(5): 299–308.
9. Poirier P, Giles TD, Bray GA, Hong Y, Stern JS, Pi-Sunyer FX, Eckel RH. (2006) Obesity and cardiovascular disease: Pathophysiology, evaluation, and effect of weight loss. *Arterioscler Thromb Vasc Biol* **26**(5): 968–976.
10. Wilson PW, D'Agostino RB, Sullivan L, Parise H, Kannel WB. (2002) Overweight and obesity as determinants of cardiovascular risk: The Framingham experience. *Arch Intern Med* **162**(16): 1867–72.
11. Wormser D, Kaptoge S, Di Angelantonio E, Wood AM, Pennells L, Thompson A, Sarwar N, Kizer JR, Lawlor DA, Nordestgaard BG, Ridker P, Salomaa V, Stevens J, Woodward M, Sattar N, Collins R, Thompson SG, Whitlock G, Danesh J. (2011) Emerging Risk Factors Collaboration. Separate and combined associations of body-mass index and abdominal adiposity with cardiovascular disease: collaborative analysis of 58 prospective studies. *Lancet* **377**(9771): 1085–95.
12. Wang TJ, Parise H, Levy D, D'Agostino RB Sr, Wolf PA, Vasan RS, Benjamin EJ. (2004) Obesity and the risk of new-onset atrial fibrillation. *JAMA* **292**(20): 2471–7.
13. Frost L, Hune LJ, Vestergaard P. (2005) Overweight and obesity as risk factors for atrial fibrillation or flutter: The Danish Diet, Cancer, and Health Study. *Am J Med* **118**(5): 489–95.
14. Kenchaiah S, Evans JC, Levy D, Wilson PW, Benjamin EJ, Larson MG, Kannel WB, Vasan RS. (2002) Obesity and the risk of heart failure. *N Engl J Med* **347**(5): 305–13.
15. Rexrode KM, Hennekens CH, Willett WC, Colditz GA, Stampfer MJ, Rich-Edwards JW, Speizer FE, Manson JE. (1997) A prospective study

of body mass index, weight change, and risk of stroke in women. *JAMA* **277**(19): 1539–45.

16. Hu G, Tuomilehto J, Silventoinen K, Sarti C, MännistöS, Jousilahti P. (2007) Body mass index, waist circumference, and waist-hip ratio on the risk of total and type-specific stroke. *Arch Intern Med* **167**(13): 1420–7.

17. Kurth T, Gaziano JM, Berger K, Kase CS, Rexrode KM, Cook NR, Buring JE, Manson JE. (2002) Body mass index and the risk of stroke in men. *Arch Intern Med* **162**(22): 2557–62.

18. Stampfer MJ, Maclure KM, Colditz GA, Manson JE, Willett WC. (1992) Risk of symptomatic gallstones in women with severe obesity. *Am J Clin Nutr* **55**(3): 652–8.

19. Turati F, Tramacere I, La Vecchia C, Negri E. (2013) A meta-analysis of body mass index and esophageal and gastric cardia adenocarcinoma. *Ann Oncol* **24**(3): 609–17.

20. Ageno W, Becattini C, Brighton T, Selby R, Kamphuisen PW. (2008) Cardiovascular risk factors and venous thromboembolism: A meta-analysis. *Circulation* **117**(1): 93–102.

21. Bacon CG, Mittleman MA, Kawachi I, Giovannucci E, Glasser DB, Rimm EB. (2003) Sexual function in men older than 50 years of age: Results from the health professionals follow-up study. *Ann Intern Med* **139**(3): 161–8.

22. Kramer H, Luke A, Bidani A, Cao G, Cooper R, McGee D. (2005) Obesity and prevalent and incident CKD: The hypertension detection and follow-up program. *Am J Kidney Dis* **46**(4): 587–94.

23. Radhakrishnan K, Ahlskog JE, Cross SA, Kurland LT, O'Fallon WM. (1993) Idiopathic intracranial hypertension (pseudotumor cerebri). Descriptive epidemiology in Rochester, Minn, 1976 to 1990. *Arch Neurol* **50**(1): 78–80.

24. Grotle M, Hagen KB, Natvig B, Dahl FA, Kvien TK. (2008) Obesity and osteoarthritis in knee, hip and/or hand: An epidemiological study in the general population with 10 years follow-up. *BMC Musculoskelet Disord* **9**: 132.

25. Felson DT, Zhang Y, Anthony JM, Naimark A, Anderson JJ. (1992). Weight loss reduces the risk for symptomatic knee osteoarthritis in women. The Framingham Study. *Ann Intern Med* **116**(7): 535–9.

26. Gortmaker SL, Must A, Perrin JM, Sobol AM, Dietz WH. (1993) Social and economic consequences of overweight in adolescence and young adulthood. *N Engl J Med* **329**(14): 1008–12.

Chapter 2

History of Bariatric Surgery

Joshua D. Pfeiffer*,‡ and Shanu N. Kothari†,§

*Minimally Invasive Bariatric Surgery and Advanced
Laparoscopy Fellowship, Department of Medical Education,
Gundersen Medical Foundation, La Crosse, WI
†Department of General and Vascular
Surgery, Gundersen Health System La Crosse, WI
‡jpfeiffer@peacehealth.org
§snkothar@gundersenhealth.org

Introduction

Throughout the 20th and 21st centuries the incidence of obesity has continued to rise and is now a worldwide health problem. Many chronic diseases, such as diabetes, hypertension and hyperlipidemia are associated with obesity. Chronic diseases now account for 84% of health care costs in the United States.[1] The most effective treatment for obesity and its associated comorbidities is bariatric surgery in its various forms. Initially a morbid, high-risk operation of last resort for patients at the extremes of obesity, bariatric surgery has become a safe, effective and proven therapy. Yet only 1% of eligible patients will have surgery. The reason for this is multifactorial, but misconceptions about the safety and efficacy of weight loss surgery by patients, health care providers, hospital administrators and insurance

---

§corresponding author.

companies accounts for much of the opposition. While efficacy and safety have improved, this field continues to evolve and advance. This evolution of bariatric surgery has been driven by surgeons adapting operations and utilizing innovation to maximize weight loss results and improvement in obesity related comorbidities, while minimizing harm to the patient. Understanding this history is essential to improve upon the decades of influential work already accomplished.

Jejunoileal Bypass (JIB)

Obesity began to capture the attention of the medical community during the first half of the 20th century, but it was not until the 1950s that surgical options for weight loss began to be explored. Dr. Viktor Henrikson is credited with the first surgical attempt at weight loss.[2,3] He anecdotally noted that some cases of bowel resection had resulted in "favorable side-effects concerning weight and intestinal function." Therefore, in 1952 he resected 105 cm of small intestine in a 32 year-old woman. The indications for surgery were not only obesity, but "constipation and something that slowed her metabolism." The short case report does not document her preoperative weight or any operative details, but the enterectomy did not result in weight loss and the patient actually gained 2 kg after 14 months. Henrikson did not consider this a failure, however, since she had improved energy, bowel function and was content with the operation. He concluded that further investigation into small bowel resection for weight loss is recommended. Meanwhile, research at the University of Minnesota was already underway and would lay the groundwork for the future of bariatric surgery.

Dr. Richard L. Varco with the help of Drs. Kremen and Linner were studying small bowel absorption in canines and the effect that controlled resection of bowel had on weight and growth.[4,5] It has been reported that Dr. Varco performed the first intestinal bypass for weight loss in 1953, but this was never published.[4] In 1954 Kremen *et al.* described their first intestinal bypass in a human patient.[5] Ninety-one cm of jejunum was anastomosed to 46 cm of ileum in an end-to-end fashion. The bypassed segment of bowel was drained into the transverse colon.

In Surgical Treatment for Obesity, Dr. Edward Mason describes his experience with small bowel bypass in the early 1950s.[6] He first attempted an end to end JIB, which did not result in any weight loss, as the patient continued to gain weight. He then performed a jejunocolic bypass (JCB) which resulted in severe diarrhea requiring revisional surgery to increase the length of functional small bowel. These and other unpublished experimentation with small bowel bypass continued sporadically through the late 1950s.

In 1963 Payne *et al.* described their experience with JCB.[7] This was initially designed as a temporary measure for the patient to achieve rapid weight loss before a second definitive operation could restore some intestinal length in order to maintain a more normal weight. Eleven patients underwent a JCB with varying results and all patients were eventually reversed or converted to a JIB. Quickly, the importance of maintaining the ileocecal valve in order to minimize the severe postoperative complications of dehydration and unrelenting diarrhea was realized. Other troubling complications of altered taste, liver failure and death were widely reported.[8,9,10] In spite of this, published reports of JCB continued until 1978.[11] However, the majority of research began to focus on optimization of the JIB.

In 1969, Payne and Dewind published their experience with JIB and described the 14 + 4 technique, where 14 inches of jejunum was anastomosed to 4 inches of terminal ileum in an end-to-side fashion.[12] The 14 + 4 procedure became a popular version of JIB due to the successful weight loss reported. However, concern arose over reflux of intestinal contents into the bypassed limb of intestine. It was thought that this reflux was responsible for some of the weight regain that patients occasionally experienced. Several techniques were described to valve the anastomosis in order to prevent reflux into the bypassed limb.[13–16]

In 1971 three different reports came out describing variations of the JIB using an end-to-end anastomosis with drainage of the bypassed section of bowel into the colon.[17–19] While reflux could still occur into the bypassed limb from the colon, the presence of anaerobic bacteria was thought to prevent absorption of nutrients. No clear advantage was ever shown between end to side or end to end anastomoses.

JIB became widely accepted as the procedure of choice for obese patients through the 1970s and an estimated 200,000 were performed in the United States alone.[4] The JIB had excellent weight loss with reports of 65–84% excess weight loss (EWL). It also had relatively low perioperative morbidity and mortality. Improvement of obesity-related comorbidities was common, including hypertension, diabetes, hyperlipidemia, reproductive problems and respiratory problems. While the perioperative risks had become accepted by physicians and the public, long-term complications of JIB began to undermine its popularity by the end of the 1970s. Diarrhea, electrolyte abnormalities, vitamin malabsorption, arthralgias, nephrolithiasis and liver failure all occurred to varying degrees. While JIB was in its height of popularity, surgeons were still searching for a better operation; one that would eliminate the metabolic complications of intestinal bypass, but still achieve weight loss and resolution of comorbidities.

Gastric Bypass

In 1965, Dr. Edward E. Mason was inspired to pursue gastric resection as a means for weight loss.[6] Dr. Wangensteen had reported that Billroth II gastrectomy for peptic ulcer disease was commonly associated with poor weight maintenance. Hearing this, Mason began experimenting with various extents of gastric resections in dogs in order to find a procedure that was not prohibitively ulcerogenic.[20] He found that a 2/3 gastric bypass achieved sufficiently low levels of acid secretion in the pouch. On May 10th, 1966 he performed the first gastric bypass on a patient who was morbidly obese and had a large incisional hernia in her lower abdomen. He performed a retrocolic loop gastrojejunostomy to the fundus of the stomach, which was approximately 20% of the original volume. The patient lost 60 pounds in 9 months and after instilling pneumoperitoneum over 6 weeks, the hernia was repaired. Mason and Ito also describe their early experience with 7 other patients who underwent a loop gastric bypass.[6] It was noted that the patients did not lose weight at a dangerous rate. One patient who weighed 125 pounds had the operation for a perforated duodenal ulcer and he had gained weight to 131 pounds at 8 months postoperative.

Mason further modified his gastric bypass in the early 1970s. He was dissatisfied with the technical difficulty of creating a gastrojejunostomy high up at the fundus and occasionally the jejunum would not reach without undue tension. He began creating a pouch of tubularized stomach and anastomosing the jejunum to it.[6] These patients tended to have difficulty with gastric emptying. In 1976, Alden modified the gastric bypass further by not dividing the stomach.[21] He simply partitioned the stomach with a staple line and performed an antecolic gastrojejunostomy. Griffen *et al.* in 1977, proposed a Roux-en-Y reconstruction of bowel in order to prevent complications of bile reflux that occurred with the loop gastrojejunostomy.[22] While this procedure had greater potential for perioperative morbidity with creation of two anastomoses, an anastomotic leak was easier to manage and less deadly, because bile and pancreatic juice had been diverted from the gastrojejunostomy.

In 1983, Torres *et al.* modified the gastric pouch so that it was created from the lesser curvature of the stomach, rather than the fundus.[23] This provided several advantages. The creation of an anastomosis on the lesser curvature was technically easier because of improved exposure and less tension on the Roux limb. There was also concern that pouches created from the fundus of the stomach were distensible and prone to dilatation and weight regain. The thicker musculature of the lesser curvature was thought to be less likely to stretch postoperatively. Concerns over distension of the gastric pouch led to additional modifications. In 1988, Salmon proposed a banded gastroplasty[24] and in 1991 Fobi described using a silastic ring to minimize pouch dilatation.[25]

Gastric bypass offered many advantages over the purely malabsorptive JIB. Diarrhea as well as liver damage is avoided, and other metabolic complications are rare. However, weight loss is lower and less durable with gastric bypass, lifelong supplementation of vitamins is still necessary and there are complications unique to the gastric bypass such as marginal ulcer and dumping syndrome.

Perioperative complications of gastrojejunostomy leak can be devastating and lethal. It was these complications that prompted Mason to find an even safer operation, even as he continued to develop the gastric bypass.

Gastroplasty

In 1971, Printen and Mason described the horizontal gastroplasty.[26] This was the first purely restrictive operation described for the management of obesity. The hope was that the weight loss seen in the gastric bypass would be duplicated by restricting intake with a small gastric pouch, but without diverting the flow of nutrients. The horizontal gastroplasty was performed by dividing the stomach from the lesser curvature towards the greater curvature and leaving a conduit for food to pass. Mason and Printen reported data on 59 patients with 6 months follow-up, but this did not result in significant weight loss.[26] This failure was attributed to a large pouch size and Mason abandoned this procedure in favor of the gastric bypass. In 1977, Gomez modified the horizontal gastroplasty to include a double staple line with reinforcement of the channel, first by a mesh collar and then by a seromuscular stitch.[27,28] These modifications were accompanied with unique complications of mesh erosion and pouch dilatation. Two reports later described removing the center staples from a TA-90 staple device so that a 1 cm channel would be created in the center of the staple line.[29,30] The horizontal gastroplasty never achieved adequate long-term weight loss, however, likely due to pouch dilatation based off of the easily distensible gastric fundus.

In 1978, Long and Collins described a gastroplasty based on the lesser curvature of the stomach.[31] A 1–2 cm stoma was created from a staple line that traveled obliquely up to the fundus, just lateral to the angle of His. This stoma was reinforced first with a polypropylene suture and later a silastic ring. Mason modified this technique and in 1980 began performing the vertical banded gastroplasty (VBG); his data were published in 1982.[32] A circular stapler was used to make a window through the lesser curvature just proximal to the incisura angularis. This window formed the outlet to the pouch and was sized with a 32 Fr bougie. A non-cutting stapler was then applied along the lesser curvature towards the angle of His so that a 50 cc pouch was created. The opening was reinforced with polypropylene mesh. Initial results showed 60% EWL at 1 year postoperative. Popularity of the VBG increased rapidly, since it was a technically easier operation to perform then the gastric bypass and did not have the complications associated with diversion of nutrients past the duodenum and proximal jejunum. However, 5 and 10-year data showed less sustained weight loss and more complications from staple line dehiscence, stomal stenosis, and mesh erosion.[33] By the late 2000s VBG was rarely being performed and many patients who had a VBG were having revisional surgery to convert their operation to a gastric bypass.[34,35]

The Magenstrasse and Mill (M&M) operation, first performed by David Johnston in 1987, was an important step in the progression of gastroplasty.[36] This was similar to the VBG in that it was based along the lesser curvature of the stomach. The circular stapler was applied more distally, at the incisura angularis just proximal to the distal branch of the nerve of Laterjet. A stapler was then applied along the lesser curve around a 32 Fr bougie and the stomach was divided. No mesh or foreign material was used in this operation. Weight loss was comparable to VBG but results were not as good as with gastric bypass. The M&M procedure would subsequently be modified to a sleeve gastrectomy in which the greater curvature of the stomach was removed. This obviated the need for the circular stapler and allowed the procedure to be done more easily laparoscopically.

Biliopancreatic Diversion (BPD) and Duodenal Switch (DS)

As gastric bypass and gastroplasty rose in popularity in the 1980s, JIB and purely malabsorptive procedures were all but abandoned in the United States. However, Scopinaro was just beginning his work on the BPD; the bariatric procedure with the most robust long-term weight loss and comorbidity resolution to date. In 1979, Scopinaro *et al.* described their initial experience with BPD.[37] This procedure combined the restrictive properties of a gastric bypass with the malabsorptive properties of intestinal bypass. A partial distal gastrectomy was performed and the duodenal stump was closed. The jejunum was then divided and reconstructed in a Roux-en-Y fashion with a 50 cm common channel and a 200 cm Roux limb that was connected to the proximal stomach. The continuous flow of bile and pancreatic juice through the biliopancreatic limb prevented the blind-loop syndrome that plagued the JIB. BPD resulted in > 75% EWL at 1 year and few patients gained this weight back.[38] Resolution of comorbidities was excellent with 98% remission of type 2 diabetes, as well as reduction of triglycerides and serum cholesterol and improvement of hypertension. These outstanding results came at a price, however, as postoperative complications could be severe. Close, lifetime follow-up was necessary to avoid and manage problems such as diarrhea, protein malnutrition, anemia, stomal ulceration, dumping syndrome and vitamin deficiencies.[39] Modification in pouch size and the lengths of intestinal bypass were varied in an attempt to minimize complications in these patients.[40]

In 1987, DeMeester *et al.* described the duodenal switch, a suprapapillary Roux-en-Y duodenojejunostomy, which was used for patients with pathologic duodenogastric reflux.[41] Lagace *et al.* modified their technique of BPD in 1990 in order to preserve the antro-pyloro-duodenal anatomy and vagus innervation along the lesser curve of the stomach.[42] This preserved gastric emptying, decreased marginal ulcer formation and prevented dumping syndrome. They stapled across the duodenum proximal to the ampulla of Vater and created a duodenoileostomy proximal to the staple line. Initial weight loss was so great in some patients that the common channel had to be revised and lengthened from 50 to 100 cm. Further, 32 of the initial 156 patients had a breakdown of the duodenal staple line with reconstitution of normal anatomic flow of nutrients by 16 months after surgery.

In 1988, Hess and Hess began their experience with the duodenal switch that would first be published in 1998.[43] They had been performing revisional surgery on patients who had failed gastro-plasty surgery for insufficient weight loss. Their preferred surgery was a revision to a BPD, but creating an anastomosis on the previously operated proximal stomach was challenging. They used the DS described by DeMeester in order to avoid this reoperative field. After good success in two patients, they began to use this as a primary procedure. They performed a partial gastrectomy of the greater curvature of the stomach around a 40 Fr bougie. They then divided the duodenum proximal to the ampulla of Vater and created an end-to-end duodenoileostomy. The ratio of the length of the common channel and alimentary limbs varied throughout their initial experience and 17 patients would eventually have a revision to both lengthen and shorten the common channel. Overall weight loss was comparable to BPD at up to 9 years follow-up.[43]

While the weight loss and resolution of comorbidities of BPD and BPD with DS are superior to any other bariatric procedure, they have not gained the popularity of the gastric bypass and restrictive procedures over the years. This is partially due to the complications after surgery as well as the technical difficulty of the surgery. While DS avoided some of the complications of BPD, the complication profile is still more severe than Roux-en-Y gastric bypass (RYGB). Through the early 1990s, banding, VBG and gastric bypass were all performed laparoscopically, but it was not until 1999 that Gagner performed the first laparoscopic DS. Now that laparoscopy has become the standard in bariatric surgery, a minority of U.S. surgeons are routinely performing DS.

Gastric Banding

The 1990s heralded the explosive rise of the laparoscopic adjustable gastric band (LAGB), but it was the initial experience with the non-adjustable gastric band and the open adjustable gastric banding that made this possible. In the mid-1970s, Wilkenson was experimenting with gastric volume reduction first in dogs, and then in humans.[44] Wilkenson and Peloso placed the first non-adjustable gastric band in 1978 in a human patient by wrapping a 2 cm strip of Marlex mesh around the proximal stomach.[45] This was followed by an array of experimentation with various forms of banding of the proximal stomach by surgeons around the world in the early 1980s.[46–50] This non-adjustable gastric volume reduction was typically created from Marlex mesh, Dacron graft, or clips. Complications of slippage and erosion were common and often required removal of the foreign body with or without revision to a different bariatric procedure. Other complications of intractable vomiting, pouch dilatation and weight regain plagued these early attempts at gastric volume restriction. Results of these early experiences in non-adjustable gastric banding showed silicone to be the best tolerated and most easily removed material.[51]

Dr. Szinicz and colleagues, of Austria, first described their experience in rabbits with an adjustable gastric band in which the inner surface of a silicone ring was lined with a balloon that could be inflated via a subcutaneous port.[52] The first reports of adjustable gastric banding in human patients were in 1985 by Hallberg and Forsell in Sweden[53] and 1986 by Kuzmak in the United States.[54] In 1993, Belachew and colleagues were the first to perform a laparoscopic placement of an adjustable gastric band.[55] This technique was quickly and universally adopted, and likely contributed to the popularity of LAGB. While a learning curve existed, it was a simpler operation to perform than a gastric bypass and had fewer perioperative complications. Similar to other restrictive procedures that preceded it, weight loss after LAGB was not as great as with gastric bypass or DS. Further weight loss occurred over 2–3 years and required consistent follow-up for band fills.[56] While the perioperative safety of the adjustable gastric bands has been well established, the long-term complications may actually occur more often. Patients who have had LAGB placement are more likely to undergo re-operation than after any other bariatric procedure.[57] Complications, such as erosions, band slippage, subcutaneous port infection and damage of the tubing, all may require operative intervention. These long-term complications combined with suboptimal weight loss and intensive lifelong follow-up have contributed to the recent decline in popularity of adjustable gastric bands. However, patients still flocked to this procedure despite these risks until another procedure came along to replace it. The emergence of the sleeve gastrectomy in the 2000s had as much or more to do with the decline in gastric banding than the gastric band's complication profile.

Sleeve Gastrectomy

The sleeve gastrectomy was first described as a "new type of gastrectomy" by Marceau *et al.* as the restrictive part of the biliopancreatic diversion.[58] This vertical gastrectomy resects 80–90% of the stomach and preserved the lesser curvature, which was turned into a sleeve-like tube, greatly restricting the capacity of the stomach. It also allows preservation of the vagal innervation of the stomach and pylorus, in order to minimize dumping syndrome. This was similar to the M&M procedure, which was first performed in 1987.[36] Regan *et al.* first proposed the advantages of staging the BPD with DS in the super morbidly obese in order to minimize perioperative morbidity and mortality.[59] Early results of staged procedures showed excellent weight loss and resolution of some comorbidities.[60,61] Subsequent second stage procedures, either DS or RYGB, were better tolerated with fewer complications,[60] although data was mixed as some studies showed no improvement in outcomes of staged vs non-staged procedures.[61] Initially, the recommendation was to proceed with the second stage surgery, but as longer-term data showed good resolution of comorbidities with sleeve gastrectomy alone, fewer patients were actually getting the second procedure.[62] Soon sleeve gastrectomy was evaluated as a stand-alone procedure.[63] The outcomes have been better than other purely restrictive procedures, but not quite as good as RYGB or DS. Early complications of sleeve gastrectomy, such as staple line leak and hemorrhage can be life threatening and difficult to manage. Late complications of stenosis, regurgitation and sleeve dilatation with weight regain are real and need continued evaluation. The optimal technique for sleeve gastrectomy is still debated and as technique is revised, outcomes may improve further. One thing is undeniable. The rise in popularity of the sleeve gastrectomy has rivaled that of the adjustable gastric band.

Minimally Invasive Techniques

Few things have influenced the growth of bariatric surgery around the world more than the implementation of laparoscopic techniques. The advantages of laparoscopy over open surgery include less pain, shorter length of stay, fewer wound complications, and a reduced rate of incisional hernia. These improvements did not come without the associated growing pains of increased perioperative complications while surgeons overcame the significant learning curve to perform these surgeries.[64]

Broadbent *et al.* were the first to report performing a laparoscopic bariatric procedure. They reported laparoscopic insertion of an adjustable gastric band on September 10, 1992.[65] This was followed up by other reports of laparoscopic gastric banding.[66] Inserting a gastric band laparoscopically was technically easier than the other commonly performed bariatric procedures, which contributed to its impressive increase in popularity.

The first laparoscopic vertical banded gastroplasty (LVBG) was performed by Hess and Hess on July 29, 1993.[67] The popularity of LVBG initially rose, especially in Europe. However, as long-term results of the VBG showed a high incidence of staple line breakdown and weight regain; the number of LVBGs being performed decreased and is now rarely performed.

The first laparoscopic Roux-en-Y gastric bypass (LRYGB) was performed in October, 1993 by Wittgrove and Clark.[68] It took longer for laparoscopy to become the preferred technique for the gastric bypass than for LAGB. This was likely due to the higher technical difficulty of LRYGB compared with LAGB and the potential perioperative complications of anastomotic leak and bleeding that were seen more frequently in early experiences with LRYGB.

The first laparoscopic DS was performed by Dr. Gagner in 1999.[69] This was even more technically difficult than the LRYGB, due to the dissection around the proximal duodenum and creation of the duodeno-ileostomy.

Robotic surgery debuted in the late 1990s and general surgeons began using robotic techniques at that same time. The first robotic-assisted bariatric procedure reported was by Talamini *et al.* in 2003.[70] They performed seven robotic-assisted gastric bypasses, but details of these procedures were not included in this report. The first totally robotic RYGB was performed by Mohr *et al.* and this was reported as a series of their first 10 totally robotic gastric bypasses.[71] Since then there have been several series of robotic gastric bypass and sleeve gastrectomy reported.[71] A clear benefit of robotic bariatric surgery has yet to be shown. The robot offers better 3D visualization, especially high in the hiatus. Also, the improved articulation and wrist-like instrumentation makes intracorporeal suturing easier and more precise. Certainly the ergonomics are improved for the surgeon who does not need to overcome torque from the abdominal wall. However, the increased cost associated with the robot and lack of sufficient evidence of clear improvement in outcomes makes the future of robotic bariatric surgery unclear.

Conclusions

Bariatric surgery has enjoyed a short but active history since the 1950s. Early pioneers such as Kremen and Mason applied basic science knowledge and observations in general surgery in the hopes of improving the overall health status of patients at the extremes of obesity. These techniques were modified and revised over the decades to improve outcomes while minimizing risk to patients. Improved technology not only influenced the course of bariatric surgery, but was, in turn, influenced greatly by the need for less invasive tools and techniques. As this field moves forward surgeons will continue to draw on lessons learned from this history to further improve surgical outcomes.

References

1. Moses H 3rd, Matheson DH, Dorsey ER *et al.* (2013) The anatomy of health care in the United States. *JAMA* **310**: 1947–1963.
2. Henrikson V. (1952) Kan tunnfarmsresektion forsvaras som terapi mot fettsot? *Nordisk Medicin* **47**: 744.

3. Henrikson V. (1994) Can small bowel resection be defended for therapy for obesity? *Obes Surg* **4**: 54–55.

4. Buchwald H, Rucker RD. (1987) The rise and fall of jejunoileal bypass. In: Nelson RL, Nyhus LM (eds), *Surgery of the Small Intestine*, pp 529–541. Appleton Century Crofts, Norwalk, CT.

5. Kremen, AJ, Linner JH, Nelson CH. (1954) An experimental evaluation of the nutritional importance of proximal and distal small intestine. *Ann Surg* **140**: 439–448.

6. Mason EE. (1981) *Surgical Treatment of Obesity.* 2nd Edition, W.B. Saunders, Philadelphia, PA.

7. Payne JH, DeWind LT, Commons RR. (1963) Metabolic observations in patients with jejunocolic shunts. *Am J Surg* **106**: 273–289.

8. Bondar GF, Pisesky W. (1967) Complications of small intestinal short-circuiting for obesity. *Arch Surg* **94**: 707–716.

9. Maxwell JG, Richards RC, AlboD Jr. (1968) Fatty degeneration of the liver after intestinal bypass for obesity. *Am J Surg* **116**: 648–652.

10. Shibata HR, Mackenzie JR, Huang S. (1971) Morphological changes of the liver following small intestinal bypass for obesity. *Arch Surg* **103**: 229–237.

11. Lavorato F, Doldi SB, Scaramella R *et al.* (1978) Evoluzione storica della terapia chirurgica della grande obesita [Historical development of the surgical treatment of gross obesity]. *Minerva Med* **69**: 3847–3857.

12. Payne JH, DeWind LT. (1969) Surgical treatment of obesity. *Am J Surg* **118**: 141–147.

13. Forestieri *et al.* (1977) Our own criteria to choose the appropriate type of jejuno-ileal bypass: A modified Payne technique. *Chir Gastroenterol* **11**: 401.

14. Forestieri P, Mosella G, De Luca L *et al.* (1978) Terapia chirurgica dell'obesita di grado elevato [Surgical treatment of severe obesity. Criteria of choice of operation. Personal technic]. *Minerva Med* **69**: 3835–3845.

15. Starkloff GB, Stothert JC, Sundaram M. (1978) Intestinal bypass: A modification. *Ann Surg* **188**: 697–700.

16. Baden H. (1971) Bypass operations in the treatment of obesity. *Ann Chir Gynaecol Fenn* **63**: 365.

17. Buchwald H, Varco RL. (1971) A bypass operation for obese hyperlipidemic patients. *Surg* **70**(1): 62–70.

18. Salmon PA. (1971) The results of small intestine bypass operations for the treatment of obesity. *Surg Gynecol Obstet* **132**: 965–979.
19. Scott HW Jr, Sandstead HH, Brill AB *et al.* (1971) Experience with a new technic of intestinal bypass in the treatment of morbid obesity. *Ann Surg* **174**: 560–572.
20. Mason EE, Ito C. (1967) Gastric bypass in obesity. *Surg Clin North Am* **47**: 1345–1351.
21. Alden JF. (1977) Gastric and jejunoileal bypass. A comparison in the treatment of morbid obesity. *Arch Surg* **112**: 799–806.
22. Griffen WO Jr, Young VL, Stevenson CC. (1977) A prospective comparison of gastric and jejunoileal bypass procedures for morbid obesity. *Ann Surg* **186**: 500–509.
23. Torres JC, Oca CF, Garrison RN. (1983) Gastric bypass: Roux-en-Y gastrojejunostomy from the lesser curvature. *South Med J* **76**: 1217–1221.
24. Salmon PA. (1988) Gastroplasty with distal gastric bypass: A new and more successful weight loss operation for the morbidly obese. *Can J Surg* **31**: 111–113.
25. Fobi M. (1991) Why the operation I prefer is silastic ring vertical gastric bypass. *Obes Surg* **1**: 423–426.
26. Printen KJ, Mason EE. (1973) Gastric surgery for relief of morbid obesity. *Arch Surg* **106**: 428–431.
27. Gomez CA. (1980) Gastroplasty in the surgical treatment of morbid obesity. *Am J Clin Nutr* **33**: 406–415.
28. Gomez CA. (1981) Gastroplasty in morbid obesity: A progress report. *World J Surg* **5**: 823–828.
29. Pace WG, Martin EW Jr, Tetirick T *et al.* (1979) Gastric partitioning for morbid obesity. *Ann Surg* **190**: 392–400.
30. Carey LC, Martin EW Jr. (1981) Treatment of morbid obesity by gastric partitioning. *World J Surg* **5**: 829–831.
31. Long M, Collins JP. (1980) The technique and early results of high gastric reduction for obesity. *Aust N Z J Surg* **50**: 146–149.
32. Mason EE. (1982) Vertical banded gastroplasty for obesity. *Arch Surg* **117**: 701–706.
33. Mason EE, Maher JW, Scott DH *et al.* (1992) Ten years of vertical banded gastroplasty for severe obesity. *Probl Gen Surg* **9**: 280–289.
34. Iannelli A, Amato D, Addeo P *et al.* (2008) Laparoscopic conversion of vertical banded gastroplasty (Mason MacLean) into Roux-en-Y gastric bypass. *Obes Surg* **18**: 43–46.

35. Marsk R, Jonas E, Gartzios H *et al.* (2009) High revision rates after laparoscopic vertical banded gastroplasty. *Surg Obes Relat Dis* **5**: 94–98.
36. Johnston D, Dachtler J, Sue-Ling HM *et al.* (2003) The Magenstrasse and Mill operation for morbid obesity. *Obes Surg* **13**: 10–16.
37. Scopinaro N, Gianetta E, Civalleri D *et al.* (1979) Bilio-pancreatic bypass for obesity: II. Initial experience in man. *Br J Surg* **66**: 618–620.
38. Scopinaro N, Adami GF, Marinari GM *et al.* (1998) Biliopancreatic diversion. *World J Surg* **22**: 936–946.
39. Scopinaro N, Gianetta E, Adami GF *et al.* (1996) Biliopancreatic diversion for obesity at eighteen years. *Surg* **119**: 261–268.
40. Scopinaro N. (2006) Biliopancreatic diversion: Mechanisms of action and long-term results. *Obes Surg* **16**: 683–689.
41. DeMeester TR, Fuchs KH, Ball CS *et al.* (1987) Experimental and clinical results with proximal end-to-end duodenojejunostomy for pathologic duodenogastric reflux. *Ann Surg* **206**: 414–426.
42. Lagacé M, Marceau P, Marceau S *et al.* (1995) Biliopancreatic diversion with a new type of Gastrectomy: Some previous conclusions revisited. *Obes Surg* **5**: 411–418.
43. Hess DS, Hess DW. (1998) Biliopancreatic diversion with a duodenal switch. *Obes Surg* **8**: 267–282.
44. Wilkinson LH. (1980) Reduction of gastric reservoir capacity. *Am J Clin Nutr* **33**: 515–517.
45. Wilkinson LH, Peloso OA. (1981) Gastric (reservoir) reduction for morbid obesity. *Arch Surg* **116**: 602–625.
46. Kolle K. (1982) Gastric banding [abstract]. *OMBI 7th Congress, Stockholm* **145**: 37.
47. Molina M, Oria HE. (1983) Gastric segmentation: A new, safe, effective, simple, readily revised and fully reversible surgical procedure for the correction of morbid obesity [abstract 15]. In: *6th Bariatric Surgery Colloquium*, Iowa City, IA.
48. Näslund E, Granström L, Stockeld D *et al.* (1994) Marlex mesh gastric banding: A 7–12 year follow-up. *Obes Surg* **4**: 269–273.
49. Frydenberg HB. (1991) Modification of gastric banding, using a fundal suture. *Obes Surg* **1**: 315–317.
50. Bashour SB, Hill RW. (1985) The gastro-clip gastroplasty: An alternative surgical procedure for the treatment of morbid obesity. *Tex Med* **81**: 36–38.

51. Steffen R. (2008) The history and role of gastric banding. *Surg Obes Relat Dis* **4**: S7–S13.

52. Szinicz G, Müller L, Erhart W *et al.* (1989) "Reversible gastric banding" in surgical treatment of morbid obesity — results of animal experiments. *Res Exp Med (Berl)* **189**: 55–60.

53. Hallberg D, Forsell O. (1985) Ballongband vid behandling av massiv oberwikt. *Svinsk Kiriurgi* **344**: 106–108.

54. Kuzmak LI. (1986) Silicone gastric banding: A simple and effective operation for morbid obesity. *Contemp Surg* **28**: 13–18.

55. Belachew M, Legrand M, Vincenti VV *et al.* (1995) Laparoscopic placement of adjustable silicone gastric band in the treatment of morbid obesity: How to do it. *Obes Surg* **5**: 66–70.

56. Shen R, Dugay G, Rajaram K *et al.* (2004) Impact of patient follow-up on weight loss after bariatric surgery. *Obes Surg* **14**: 514–519.

57. Suter M, Calmes JM, Paroz A *et al.* (2006) A 10-year experience with laparoscopic gastric banding for morbid obesity: High long-term complication and failure rates. *Obes Surg* **16**: 829–835.

58. Marceau P, Biron S, Bourque RA *et al.* (1993) Biliopancreatic diversion with a new type of gastrectomy. *Obes Surg* **3**: 29–35.

59. Regan JP, Inabnet WB, Gagner M *et al.* (2003) Early experience with two-stage laparoscopic Roux-en-Y gastric bypass as an alternative in the super-super obese patient. *Obes Surg* **13**: 861–864.

60. Silecchia G, Boru C, Pecchia A *et al.* (2006) Effectiveness of laparoscopic sleeve gastrectomy (first stage of biliopancreatic diversion with duodenal switch) on co-morbidities in super-obese high-risk patients. *Obes Surg* **16**: 1138–1144.

61. Cottam D, Qureshi FG, Mattar SG *et al.* (2006) Laparoscopic sleeve gastrectomy as an initial weight loss procedure for high-risk patients with morbid obesity. *Surg Endosc* **20**: 859–863.

62. Brethauer SA, Hammel JP, Schauer PR. Systematic review of sleeve gastrectomy as staging and primary bariatric procedure. *Surg Obes Relat Dis* 2009; **5**:469–75.

63. Gumbs AA, Gagner M, Dakin G *et al.* (2007) Sleeve gastrectomy for morbid obesity. *Obes Surg* **17**: 962–969.

64. Schauer PR, Ikramuddin S. (2001) Laparoscopic surgery for morbid obesity. *Surg Clin North Am* **81**: 1145–1179.

65. Broadbent R, Tracey M, Harrington P. (1993) Laparoscopic gastric banding: A preliminary report. *Obes Surg* **3**: 63–67.

66. Belachew M, Legrand M, Jacquet N. (1993) Laparoscopic placement of adjustable silicone gastric banding in the treatment of morbid obesity: An animal model experimental study: A video film: A preliminary report [abstract 5]. *Obes Surg* **3**: 140.

67. Hess DW, Hess DS. (1994) Laparoscopic vertical banded gastroplasty with complete transection of the staple-line. *Obes Surg* **4**: 44–46.

68. Wittgrove AC, Clark GW. (2000) Laparoscopic gastric bypass, Roux-en-Y-500 patients: Technique and results, with 3–60 month follow-up. *Obes Surg* **10**: 233–239.

69. Ren CJ, Patterson E, Gagner M. (2000) Early results of laparoscopic biliopancreatic diversion with duodenal switch: A case series of 40 consecutive patients. *Obes Surg* **10**: 514–523.

70. Talamini MA, Chapman S, Horgan S *et al.* (2003) Academic Robotics Group. A prospective analysis of 211 robotic-assisted surgical procedures. *Surg Endosc* **17**: 1521–1524.

71. Mohr CJ, Nadzam GS, Curet MJ. (2005) Totally robotic Roux-en-Y gastric bypass. *Arch Surg* **140**: 779–786.

Chapter 3

Roux-en-Y Gastric Bypass: Indications, Procedures and Outcomes

Umer I. Chaudhry* and Dean J. Mikami*,†

*Center for Minimally Invasive Surgery, The Ohio State University
Wexner Medical Center, Columbus, OH
†dean.mikami@osumc.edu

Introduction and Indications

Mason and Ito developed the first gastric bypass in 1966.[1] Instead of a Roux-en-Y anastomosis, this original operation had a loop gastrojejunostomy between the proximal gastric pouch and the proximal jejunum. It was not until 1977, that Griffen and colleagues introduced the Roux-en-Y reconstruction,[2] which allowed for excellent weight loss while decreasing the incidence of bile reflux. Since then, several iterations of the Roux-en-Y gastric bypass (RYGB) have been described. Currently, RYGB is the most commonly performed bariatric procedure in the U.S., although sleeve gastrectomy is quickly gaining in popularity and may surpass RYGB in the near future.

Many believe RYGB to be the gold-standard weight loss operation and employ it as a reference when comparing results of other bariatric surgeries. RYGB is considered a restrictive, as well as a

---

†Corresponding author.

malabsorptive bariatric procedure. The restriction is achieved by dividing the proximal stomach to create a small gastric pouch (approximately 30 ml) with a narrow outlet, and the malabsorptive element is introduced by bypassing the distal stomach (gastric remnant), the entire duodenum, and a 40 to 50 cm segment of proximal jejunum. Bowel continuity is re-established with the creation of gastrojejunal and jejunojejunal anastomoses. The length of the Roux limb can be varied anywhere from 75 to 150 cm, with longer lengths providing a more extensive malabsorptive component. We routinely fashion our Roux limb to be approximately 150 cm in length. Roux limbs longer than 150 cm are considered experimental and may not be covered by insurance. However, the length of the biliopancreatic limb can be manipulated to achieve a Roux limb of 150 cm and a common channel of 75 to 125 cm, which can also provide a more robust malabsorptive element to the operation.

Indications for RYGB are similar to other bariatric procedures and as outlined in the 1991 National Institute of Health consensus criteria for weight loss surgery.[3] Usually, patients are eligible for RYGB if their body mass index (BMI) is 40 kg/m^2 or greater, or if their BMI is between 35–40 kg/m^2 and accompanied by an obesity related medical comorbidity, such as diabetes, hypertension, obstructive sleep apnea, or gastroesophageal reflux disease.

Procedure

Typically, the operating surgeon stands on the patient's right side and the first-assistant on the left. An additional assistant is positioned at the foot of the bed and operates the camera. We prefer to gain peritoneal access via the Veress needle technique at Palmer's point. Alternatively, access can also be gained using the optical trocar technique, a Hassan cutdown technique, or any other method that the surgeon is comfortable performing. Once pneumoperitoneum is established to 15 mm Hg, working trocars are placed under direct visualization. Placement of port sites varies with the personal preference of the surgeon. Normally, a 12 mm camera port is placed in the midline and both sides of the abdominal wall are used for placement of working ports. We favor a 5 and a 15 mm port on the right side, and a 5 and a 12 mm port on the left side.

The operation is started by retracting the omentum and transverse colon superiorly, which allows for visualization of the ligament of Treitz. The small bowel is traced 40–50 cm distally from the ligament of Treitz and divided with a laparoscopic 6 cm linear stapler (2.5 mm staple height). The mesentery is divided further with a 6 cm linear stapler (2.0 mm staple height) to lengthen it. We prefer to mark the Roux limb with a blue penrose drain, which permits easy identification and helps avoid a Roux-en-O reconstruction. The jejunojejunostomy between the biliopancreatic limb and the Roux limb is created by tracing the Roux limb 150 cm distally, where a single stay suture is placed at the antimesenteric borders to align the two limbs, with the stapled end of the biliopancreatic limb positioned to the right of the Roux limb. Enterotomies are made with an energy device and the anastomosis is created with a laparoscopic 6 cm linear stapler (2.5 mm staple height). We also prefer to close the enterotomy with a linear stapler. Alternatively, the defect can be closed with an absorbable or non-absorbable suture in a running or simple interrupted fashion. Any minor bleeding at the staple lines is controlled with laparoscopic clips. A single 2-0 non-absorbable stitch is placed between the stapled end of the biliopancreatic limb and the Roux limb (Brolin stitch) to prevent kinking and subsequent obstruction. The mesenteric defect is then closed using a running 2-0 non-absorbable suture to prevent internal herniation.

For the creation of the gastric pouch and subsequent gastrojejunostomy, the patient is placed in a steep reverse Trendelenburg position. The anesthesiologist is asked to remove any gastric or esophageal tubes if they have been inserted during the beginning of the case. We prefer to use a Nathanson liver retractor in the subxiphoid space to retract the left lateral segment of the liver to gain adequate exposure. Hiatal hernia, if present, is repaired anteriorly with 0 weight non-absorbable sutures. The pars flaccida of the gastrohepatic ligament is then opened bluntly and the descending branches of the left gastric artery are divided with a laparoscopic 4.5 cm linear stapler (2.0 mm staple height). Care is taken to avoid injury to an anomalous left hepatic artery, if present.

Several techniques are available for the creation of gastrojejunostomy. We prefer to use a 25 mm circular stapler to create an end-to-side anastomosis. Thus, a distal gastrotomy is created in the body of the stomach with an energy device and the anvil from a 25 mm circular stapler is introduced into the peritoneal cavity via the right-sided 15 mm port site. (We typically use a 4.5 mm staple height for males and a 3.5 mm staple height for females.) The anvil is then placed through the distal gastrotomy and brought out via a second gastrotomy made 3–4 cm from the gastroesophageal junction. A reticulating Maryland grasper can be helpful during this step of the procedure. The distal gastrotomy is closed with a 6 cm linear stapler (3.5 mm staple height). (Alternatively, the anvil can be placed by mouth after the gastric pouch has been constructed.)

A 20–30 ml gastric pouch is created around the anvil using a laparoscopic linear stapler. The first staple line is made transversely and the subsequent staple lines are created longitudinally towards the angle of His. Complete division of the stomach is verified. Next, the Roux limb is brought up to the gastric pouch in an antecolic-antegastric fashion for the creation of the gastrojejunal anastomosis. Additional 3–4 cm of the Roux limb mesentery can be divided to facilitate this step of the procedure. The staple line of the Roux limb is opened with an energy device and the hammer part of the circular stapler is inserted into the peritoneal cavity via the 15 mm port site and advanced into the lumen of the proximal Roux limb. The spike of the stapler is deployed through the antimesenteric surface and connected to the anvil in the gastric pouch. The alignment is checked and an end-to-side gastrojejunostomy is then created. The overhang of the Roux limb is divided with a linear staler and a 2-0 absorbable suture is placed at the corner of the anastomosis to reduce tension.

Integrity of the gastrojejunal anastomosis is checked by clamping the proximal Roux limb and performing an intraoperative endoscopy. The anastomosis should be widely patent with no evidence of bleeding. Additionally, there should be no air bubbles seen with the anastomosis immersed under saline to suggest a leak. We do not routinely place nasogastric tubes or leave drains adjacent to the gastrojejunal anastomosis. Trocar sites of 10 mm or greater are closed with 0 weight absorbable sutures using a suture passer device. The wounds were copiously irrigated and the skin is closed in two layers.

Outcomes

With the advent of minimally invasive techniques in the 1980s, bariatric surgery has experienced a new renaissance. Wittgrove and colleagues published the first series of laparoscopic RYGB in 1994 and helped usher in this new era.[4] Outcomes from laparoscopic surgery are unparalleled compared to open technique, with a significant decrease in wound complications and ventral hernia formation.[5] Currently, vast majority of RYGB are performed laparoscopically and the open technique is becoming more and more extinct.

Patients who undergo RYGB typically experience a percent excess weight loss (%EWL) of 60%–70% at 2 years, with resolution of comorbidities seen in 70%–95% of the individuals.[6, 7] Thirty-day mortality is usually reported to be less than 0.5%, and attributable mostly to fatal pulmonary embolisms or sepsis secondary to anastomotic leaks. Several meta-analyses have confirmed these results.[6–8] In the latest meta-analysis by Chang and colleagues,[7] which analyzed 37 randomized clinical trials, the 30-day mortality rate was 0.08% and the rate after 30-day was observed to be 0.39%. The 30-day complication rate was reported to be 21%. The %EWL at 1- and 2-years was 72% and 74%, respectively. In regards to resolution of comorbidities, Chang *et al.* reported remission rates of 95%, 81%, 80% and 95% for diabetes, hypertension, dyslipidemia and obstructive sleep apnea, respectively.

Complications from RYGB can be divided into early and late, depending on the time of presentation. Some early or perioperative complications include bleeding, anastomotic leaks and venous thromboembolism (VTE). The incidence of gastrointestinal bleeding has been reported in up to 4% of the patients.[9] Anastomotic leaks can be seen in up to 5% of the patients and represent one of the most feared and potentially devastating complications.[10] The overall incidence of VTE ranges from 0.1 to 3.8%,[11] albeit the prevalence of asymptomatic VTE remains unknown. There is no consensus on appropriate VTE prophylaxis in patients undergoing bariatric surgery. However, most surgeons routinely use some form of prophylaxis. High index of suspicion is necessary to diagnose and treat these complications before they become fatal, as morbidly obese patients do not elicit the same symptoms as normal weight patients.

Late complications can include intestinal obstruction from an internal hernia or adhesions, anastomotic stricture, or marginal ulceration, although these can also present early in the postoperative period. Incidence of internal hernias after laparoscopic RYGB is estimated to be 3%–5%,[12,13] and can be devastating if not diagnosed early. Internal hernias typically occur at three potential spaces: (1) Mesenteric defect at the jejunojejunostomy, (2) Petersen's defect and (3) transverse colon mesenteric defect in cases of retrocolic Roux limb. Marginal ulcers are common after RYGB and can be seen in 1%–16% of the patients.[14,15] Several risk factors, including local ischemia, foreign body reaction, large pouch size, gastro-gastric fistula, h pylori infection, smoking and non-steroidal anti-inflammatory medication use have been implicated in the formation of marginal ulcers. Anastomotic strictures are also common and can occur as early as 3 to 4 week after RYGB. The incidence is reported to be anywhere from 5% to 27%.[16] Although the etiology is unclear, local ischemia, recurrent marginal ulcers, tension at the anastomosis, circular stapler (vs linear) and stapler size (21 mm vs 25 mm), have been linked with anastomotic strictures.

Significant weight loss recidivism can be seen in up to 20% of the patients at long-term follow-up.[17] This weight regain can have important health consequence including recurrence of obesity-related medical comorbidities. Recently, Coleman et al. published three-year weight loss outcomes from the bariatric registry of a large intergraded healthcare system.[18] Fifty-eight percent of the 20,296 patients had undergone RYGB and greater than 50% were ethnic minorities. The median %EWL at 1-year was reported to be 67%. However, at

3 years, the median %EWL had decreased to 59%. Additionally, findings from the study showed that gender plays an important role in outcomes, as women experienced a significantly higher %EWL than men (61% vs 55%) at 3 years. Furthermore, race also has an effect on outcomes, as Caucasian patients seemed to benefit the greatest from RYGB with %EWL of approximately 63% at 3 years, compared to 59% for Hispanics and 56% for African–Americans.

Small percentage of the patients experience weight loss recidivism due to surgery related factors, such as loss of restriction due to gastric pouch and/or stoma dilation or formation of a gastro-gastric fistula. Majority of the patients, however, experience weight regain due to lifestyle changes, such as dietary non-compliance or physical inactivity. Ideally, these patients showed be treated with nutritional and lifestyle counseling, as operative intervention is rarely successful. It is vital for the patients to understand that bariatric surgery represents a tool to assist with weight loss and must be combined with life-long lifestyle changes to achieve durable results.

References

1. Mason EE, Ito C. (1967) Gastric bypass in obesity. *Surg Clin North Am* **47**(6): 1345–1351.
2. Griffen WO, Jr., Young VL, Stevenson CC. (1977) A prospective comparison of gastric and jejunoileal bypass procedures for morbid obesity. *Ann Surg* **186**(4): 500–509.
3. NIH Conference. (1991) Gastrointestinal surgery for severe obesity. Consensus Development Conference Panel. *Ann Intern Med* **115**(12): 956–961.
4. Wittgrove AC, Clark GW, Tremblay LJ. (1994) Laparoscopic gastric bypass, roux-en-Y: Preliminary report of five cases. *Obes Surg* **4**(4): 353–357.
5. Reoch J, Mottillo S, Shimony A *et al.* Safety of laparoscopic vs open bariatric surgery: A systematic review and meta-analysis. *Arch Surg* **146**(11): 1314–1322.
6. Buchwald H, Avidor Y, Braunwald E *et al.* Bariatric surgery: A systematic review and meta-analysis. *JAMA* **292**(14): 1724–1737.

7. Chang SH, Stoll CR, Song J *et al.* (2014) The effectiveness and risks of bariatric surgery: An updated systematic review and meta-analysis, 2003–2012. *JAMA Surg* **149**(3): 275–287.

8. Colquitt JL, Picot J, Loveman E *et al.* (2009) Surgery for obesity. *Cochrane Database Syst Rev* (2):CD003641.

9. Nguyen NT, Longoria M, Chalifoux S *et al.* (2004) Gastrointestinal hemorrhage after laparoscopic gastric bypass. *Obes Surg* **14**(10): 1308–1312.

10. Fernandez AZ, Jr., DeMaria EJ, Tichansky DS *et al.* (2004) Experience with over 3,000 open and laparoscopic bariatric procedures: Multivariate analysis of factors related to leak and resultant mortality. *Surg Endosc* **18**(2): 193–197.

11. Escalante-Tattersfield T, Tucker O, Fajnwaks P *et al.* (2008) Incidence of deep vein thrombosis in morbidly obese patients undergoing laparoscopic Roux-en-Y gastric bypass. *Surg Obes Relat Dis* **4**(2): 126–130.

12. Garza E, Jr., Kuhn J, Arnold D, *et al.* (2004) Internal hernias after laparoscopic Roux-en-Y gastric bypass. *Am J Surg* **188**(6): 796–800.

13. Iannelli A, Facchiano E, Gugenheim J. (2006) Internal hernia after laparoscopic Roux-en-Y gastric bypass for morbid obesity. *Obes Surg* **16**(10): 1265–1271.

14. Huang CS, Forse RA, Jacobson BC *et al.* (2003) Endoscopic findings and their clinical correlations in patients with symptoms after gastric bypass surgery. *Gastrointest Endosc* **58**(6): 859–866.

15. Schauer PR, Ikramuddin S, Gourash W *et al.* (2000) Outcomes after laparoscopic Roux-en-Y gastric bypass for morbid obesity. *Ann Surg* **232**(4): 515–529.

16. Ryskina KL, Miller KM, Aisenberg J *et al.* (2010) Routine management of stricture after gastric bypass and predictors of subsequent weight loss. *Surg Endosc* **24**(3): 554–560.

17. Karmali S, Brar B, Shi X *et al.* (2013) Weight recidivism post-bariatric surgery: A systematic review. *Obes Surg* **23**(11): 1922–1933.

18. Coleman KJ, Huang YC, Hendee F *et al.* (2014) Three-year weight outcomes from a bariatric surgery registry in a large integrated healthcare system. *Surg Obes Relat Dis* **10**(3): 396–403.

Chapter 4

Biliopancreatic Diversion and Duodenal Switch: Indications, Procedure and Outcomes

Patrick Fei* and Fernando Bonanni[†,‡]

*Abington Jefferson Health,
1200 Old York Road, Abington PA 19001
† The Institute for Metabolic and Bariatric Surgery,
Abington Jefferson Health, 1200 Old York Road,
Abington PA 19001

Introduction

The condition of obesity is often discussed as occurring in epidemic proportions and has become the major health issue in the world surpassing starvation.[1] In the current healthcare environment, the added burden of cost containment necessitates treatment options that result in durable success, minimal recidivism and low rates of complication and mortality. Since the 1950's, metabolic surgeons have sought to apply the most appropriate surgical principles to address the problem of obesity; the history of these operations is summarized in an earlier chapter. As understanding of the problem of obesity and its metabolic consequences has evolved, so too have the operations performed to address them.

‡ Corresponding author.

Biliopancreatic diversion with duodenal switch (BPD/DS) is a complex operation that requires close follow-up by the metabolic team and full cooperation by the patient for optimal results. BPD/DS offers superior results in excess weight loss,[2,3] sustained resolution of diabetes of ≥90%,[4] the most significant impact on comorbid disease,[3] the ability to modify to a patient's specific profile, low short- and long-term complication rates,[5,6] the lowest revision rate for weight regain[2,6] and a low rate of nutritional derangements in the compliant patient.[6]

Background

There are four major bariatric procedures available to the patient: Adjustable gastric banding, vertical sleeve gastrectomy, gastric bypass and BPD/DS, all of which are preferentially done laparoscopically. Bariatric procedures are based on the principles of *restriction* and *diversion*. In restriction, a gastric reservoir is fashioned into a small pouch to limit caloric volume, which can be accomplished through either band placement (adjustable and reversible) or resection/division. The restrictive component of bariatric procedures depends on satiety as well as alteration to levels of the hunger hormone ghrelin. Satiety is also influenced by the stretch receptors in the stomach lining.[7]

Diversion, also often referred to as *malabsorption,* is based on exclusion of the proximal intestinal tract (duodenum) and stimulation of the distal intestinal tract (ileum). The result is the diversion of calories and a change in the nature of the hormones that control the metabolism of carbohydrates and other substrates. This is referred to as the *entero-insulin axis.*[8–11] Through this process, insulin becomes more abundant, efficient and effective. Diversion impacts both hunger and the nature of absorption: What is absorbed, where it is absorbed, how it is absorbed, how much is absorbed and over what duration. Restriction and diversion are more effective when used in combination.

Development of BPD/DS

In the mid to late 1970s, Scopinaro developed BPD to address the recidivism and poor results in super morbidly obese (SMO) patients following the gastric bypass procedure, as well as the high failure rates of the then available restrictive procedures.[12] Scopinaro also designed BPD to be a safer malabsorptive alternative to jejunoileal bypass. BPD induces a more controlled malabsorption in a compliant patient and because of the absence of the long bypassed loop, it is also free of the potential side effects caused by bacterial overgrowth associated with the jejunoileal bypass.[13] Scopinaro applied physiological principles that decreased food absorption and, at the same time, preserved relatively normal eating patterns without imposing food aversion. The intention was to make weight loss a function of absorption and less an aversion to eating. The BPD employed a significant reduction of the gastric volume through distal gastrectomy with closure of the duodenal stump. The diversionary aspect of this procedure involves creating a long Roux-en-Y reconstruction where the entero-enterostomy is constructed 50 cm proximal to the ileocecal valve. The gastroenterostomy is located 250 cm from the ileocecal valve, creating a 250 cm alimentary limb. Cholecystectomy often accompanied the procedure.

At first the Scopinaro BPD was used as revision surgery for failed restrictive procedures. It soon proved to be a useful primary operation for obese patients. Its emphasis on malabsorption was found to be highly effective in weight loss maintenance and resolution of comorbid disease. The resolution of diabetes was significant, rapid and long lasting, which was attributed to duodenal exclusion and distal small bowel stimulation.[14] At 10-year follow-up, 90% of patients had an excess body weight (EBW) loss of >50%; failure rate was <1%. Resolution of comorbid disease in over 2000 patients was significant, with 100% resolution of noninsulin-dependent diabetes mellitus (NIDDM) and only four relapses of hyperglycemia not requiring treatment 14 years the procedure.[12]

Problems with BPD stemmed primarily from the distal gastrectomy and gastro jejunostomy components of the operation. Long-term complications included marginal ulceration, protein deficiency and iron and calcium deficiency.[13,15] Complications from June 1984 to July 2003 decreased as experience increased. Operative mortality steadily decreased to less than 0.5%. General complications decreased to 0.2%–0.4%; major surgical complications decreased to

1.2%–1.4% and consisted of intraperitoneal bleeding, wound dehiscence and wound infection.[16]

Framework for BPD/DS

In 1988, Hess and Hess combined Scopinaro's BPD and DeMeester's duodenal switch (DS) to create a hybrid operation with the intention of reducing complications seen in the traditional BPD. In 1987, DeMeester *et al.* had reported on the DS for bile reflux, which was developed as an alternative to Roux-en-Y gastrojejunostomy.[17] To incorporate this into the BPD, a vertical gastric sleeve was created instead of a gastric pouch with distal gastrectomy as Scopinaro had described. An ileal anastomosis was made onto the first part of the duodenum, thus preserving pyloric function and eliminating small bowel exposure to gastric acids. Hess intended to combine the adequate weight loss and resolution of diabetes provided by BPD with the reduction of marginal ulceration and dumping as described by DeMeester. Postoperative results included rare marginal ulcer, decreased dumping syndrome and less iron and calcium malabsorption.

In 1998, Hess and Hess reported on the first 440 patients who had undergone this new procedure, the BPD/DS. None of these patients had undergone previous bariatric surgery; 41% were considered SMO (BMI > 50). By 24 months postoperatively, there was an average maximum weight loss of 80% excess weight; this trend continued at a 70% level for 8 years. Two perioperative deaths occurred (massive pulmonary embolism; respiratory arrest with bilateral bronchial obstruction). Major complications occurred in approximately 9% of patients. There were 17 revisions (8 for low protein and excessive weight loss, 7 for inadequate weight loss and 2 for excessive diarrhea). All 36 type-2 diabetic patients were able to discontinue medication.[18]

In 2005, Hess, Hess and Oakley reported on their continued experience of over 1400 cases, of which 159 were reoperations from other failed procedures.[6] They reported an overall EBW loss of 75%

after 10 years and over 90% resolution of NIDDM. The revision rate was 3.7% and the reversal rate was 0.61%. The authors described measuring the small bowel stretched between instruments. After measuring the total length of small bowel, the alimentary limb was created at 40% of the total length (as opposed to using a fixed 250 cm in the Scopinaro BPD). This was done to address the variability in small bowel lengths between different patients. The common channel was created using 10% of the total bowel length measured proximally from the ileocecal valve. As a result, the average common channel limb lengths varied from 75–125 cm but were similarly proportional in each patient.

In the first 1300 patients, 98% of the type-2 diabetics became euglycemic a few weeks postoperatively. Sleep apnea was cured. Hypertension resolved in most patients, with medication usage reduced in others. Hyperventilation syndrome of obesity, hypercholesterolemia and other comorbidities were also corrected or improved.

Principles of BPD/DS

The goals of a successful BPD/DS include adequate weight loss, minimal recidivism and minimal consequences to nutritional derangements. The technical principles involved can be summarized as follows:

Principle 1

The entire small bowel must be measured; the common channel created is 10% of this length while the alimentary limb is 40% of the entire small bowel length. These percentages reflect the optimal lengths for adequate absorption of necessary nutrients while diverting sufficient calories to obtain weight loss. After adaptation, the length of the common channel maintains weight loss in compliant patients. These percentages are the key to accounting for variable bowel lengths (as different as 345 cm to 1140 cm as described by Hess and Hess).

Principle 2

The measurements must be consistent for reproducible results. This can be assured by stretching the bowel fully and measuring along the antimesenteric border.[19] There can be considerable differences in small bowel lengths within the same patient, depending on the conditions of the bowel when measured.

Principle 3

The sleeved stomach must be small (100–120 ml) with an adequate anastomosis for emptying. However, a standard-sized vertical gastric sleeve (used in stand-alone procedures) should not be used in conjunction with severe diversion. If stomal outlet obstruction occurs, the overly restrictive component will limit the patient's ability to eat adequate protein in relation to the amount of diversion occurring downstream, resulting in dangerous hypoproteinemia. Similarly, an overly shortened common channel will result in worse nutritional difficulties and their sequelae.

Principle 4

Compliance with supplementation, diet and extensive life-long follow-up are essential for success after BPD/DS. In the authors' experience, it is not uncommon for patients to begin to feel well after weight loss and then start neglecting these principles, leading to undesirable consequences.

Diabetes and the Entero-Insulin Axis

An estimated 90% of diabetic patients are overweight, with an exponential increase in risk with severity.[20] The diversion of BPD/DS is thought to impact directly on NIDDM through the entero-insulin axis by the manipulation of gut hormones (ghrelin and incretins). Incretins are stimulated by nutrients to cause both proliferation of the pancreatic B cells as well as inhibition of their regression, effectively improving sensitivity to insulin and inhibiting gastric emptying; the result is a decrease in food intake.

Ghrelin, produced mostly in the gastric fundus, is secreted as a potent appetite stimulant. It also has pro-diabetic effects by suppression of insulin. Ghrelin directly opposes insulin action, stimulates counter-regulatory hormones, down-regulates energy expenditure and preserves body fat.

Diversion by bariatric surgery changes the nature of incretins secreted by the gut in favor of efficient use of insulin through increased sensitivity and enhanced insulin production. By excluding the duodenum and stimulating the distal small intestine, carbohydrate metabolism becomes more efficient. Gastric inhibitory peptide (GIP) is down-regulated at the beta-cell level, but is more effective when excluding the duodenum. GIP is secreted by the duodenal K cells after digestion of fat and carbohydrates; it increases B-cell sensitivity.[8,14]

Distal stimulation of the small intestine stimulates insulin secretion through increased production of glucagon-like peptide (GLP). Rapid delivery of undigested nutrients in the small bowel up-regulate the gut L cells to stimulate insulin regulation, delay gastric emptying, induce glycogenesis and inhibit glucagon.[8,14] There is substantial evidence that suggests a direct correlation with insulin resistance and obesity in the metabolic syndrome (increased triglycerides, decreased high density lipoprotein, hypertension, increased fasting blood sugar and obesity).[21]

The overall impact on diabetes and mortality after bariatric surgery varies depending on the resultant weight loss and degree of intestinal diversion.[22] Results for gastric banding, sleeve gastrectomy, gastric bypass and BPD/DS respectively are as follows (%): Excess weight loss 38, 49, 70, 84 [23]; remission of type-2 diabetes mellitus 47, 66, 83, 99.[24] Surgical weight loss procedures have long been known to impact NIDDM through mechanisms related to excess fat energy including decreased caloric intake, decreased intestinal absorption of fat and loss of adipose tissue resulting in less insulin resistance. These contribute to the restoration of the acute insulin response (beta cell sensitivity). Metabolic changes promoting increased insulin sensitivity begin immediately and have been detected as early as 3 weeks postoperatively.[8] Other mechanisms include decreased ghrelin (pro-diabetic hormone/hunger resistance and the entero-insulin axis), duodenal exclusion (<GIP) and distal small bowel stimulation (>GLP).

Specifically, BPD/DS results in greater weight loss by combining sleeve restriction with significantly greater diversion. Greater excess weight loss results in less total body fat, less intestinal absorption of fat and an overall decrease in calories. The gastric sleeve produces less total gastric volume with a greater impact on ghrelin, which affects appetite stimulation and insulin resistance. BPD/DS excludes the duodenum, which results in the down-regulation of GIP at the beta-cell level. Results of >90% short- and long-term resolution of NIDDM with significantly improved parameters in NIDDM have been reported.[5,6]

Advantages/Indications

Preservation of the pylorus is the natural mechanism that controls nutrient flow into the intestinal tract. It results in slower gastric emptying and serves as a natural defense against dumping and ulcers. Pyloric preservation has the lowest rate of recidivism and the greatest impact on diabetes mellitus. With adjustments to the length of the common channel and the size of the vertical sleeve, it is conceivable that any obese patient is a candidate for BPD/DS.

In SMO patients (BMI > 50 and/or >150 lbs EBW), BPD/DS has proven to have better short- and long-term results.[25] Patients who are not at least 150 lbs overweight or have a BMI < 50 have a greater risk of excessive weight loss and malnutrition, even when they are compliant. In these circumstances BPD/DS is still the most adjustable surgical option. It is not necessary to offer a standard common channel (75–100 cm) and the available length of the common channel can be adjusted to avoid excessive bowel movements and excessive weight loss. In addition, the surgeon can adjust the size of the sleeve and alter the impact of the restriction that is added to the diversional weight loss. This author offers up to a 150 cm common channel, depending on clinical parameters specific to each patient.

Other candidates for BPD/DS include patients with severe or poorly controlled NIDDM over 10 years and patients who are on chronic anticoagulants who are at increased risk of bleeding from the gastrojejunostomy of the gastric bypass. Patients who are taking chronic ulcerogenic drugs, such as NSAIDS and steroids, who in the past would have been offered gastric banding or the vertical sleeve, would have the normal physiologic barriers to ulcers in the sleeve portion of the BPD/DS and benefit from a modified diversion. Common channels <100 cm or <10% of the bowel length are more likely to result in malnutrition and excessive bowel movements.[19]

The obvious advantages of the BPD/DS are the greater weight loss overall, the success in SMO patients and the impressive resolution of NIDDM. Other advantages of BPD/DS over gastric bypass and other traditional surgical weight loss procedures include absence of a foreign body, intact pylorus, elimination of dumping and no increased risk for ulcers. BPD/DS patients can adopt more normal eating patterns after adaptation to volume and content. Since dumping is not usually an issue, food ingested with higher glucose or fructose concentrations in moderation will not cause postprandial hypoglycemic symptoms. Patients with esophagogastric pathology (peptic ulcer disease, gastric dysplasia, gastric polyps and family history of gastric cancer) are not left with a gastric remnant that cannot be surveyed.

Disadvantages of the BPD/DS

The greatest challenge to the surgeon is adopting and mastering the steep learning curve, which may result in initial higher technical complication rates and longer operative times.[26] Proctoring can help address both of these issues. Committed surgeons who already perform gastric bypass can transition relatively seamlessly into these techniques. Equally as intimidating and prohibitive is the implementation of a robust postoperative follow-up program addressing the specific needs of these patients.

Preoperative Evaluation and Preparation

Since the early 2000s, it became increasingly evident that success in surgical weight loss depends on a comprehensive multidisciplinary program. Through the Centers of Excellence (COE) programs emerged models for a multidisciplinary approach, including medical work-up, psychological evaluation, nutritional evaluation, preoperative education regarding postoperative expectations, behavior modification, physical activity and support required for success.[27] Special attention needs to be paid to the patient's ability to comply with a rigorous postoperative regimen and the patient's ability to commit both emotionally and financially to the process.

Psychiatric evaluation

Psychiatric evaluation is critical for the BPD/DS patient. In our experience, the following psychological criteria must be met: (1) No recent or present suicidal ideation, (2) no active substance abuse, (3) no psychosis, (4) reasonable understanding for the postoperative regimen, (5) understanding of the behavioral modification techniques required for success, (6) adequate psychosocial support and (7) realistic expectations. Patients lost to follow-up who are not compliant are at risk for serious nutritional deficit, neurologic and social consequences and ultimately, death.

Nutritional consultation

Nutritional evaluation and consultation is the center piece to success for all surgical weight loss procedures, especially BPD/DS. The patient must be educated on the expected postoperative diet regimen, with an emphasis on learning the potential consequences of nutritional deficiency if they are not compliant. The patient will also learn how to schedule supplements and meals as a priority for success. Nutritional cornerstones include the following: High-protein, low-fat diet (80 g protein per day), adequate hydration, vitamin deficiency evaluation and mechanical eating (portion control, avoidance of liquid calories, nighttime eating, drinking with eating). Pitfalls include avoiding the following: Soda, caffeine, tobacco, alcohol, spicy food, fats and carbohydrates such as pretzels, crackers and candy. These can worsen symptoms of flatulence and steatorrhea.

In our experience, the most common danger for the BPD/DS patient has been self-induced malnutrition from lack of compliance. Patients are sometimes deceived by their weight loss, increased energy and euphoria from the initial weight loss. Patients who underestimate their nutritional responsibilities begin to see the consequences after 9 months to 1 year. The most common initial symptoms are fatigue and peripheral edema. After protein malnutrition manifests along with other nutritional derangements, achieving homeostasis can take an additional 9 months to 1 year.

Diversion in the beginning is extensive and can result in significant nutritional issues, including: Protein deficiency, fat-soluble vitamin deficiencies (ADEK), iron deficiency, calcium deficiency and B-complex deficiencies.[28] These deficiencies in combination can cause a number of complications that include peripheral edema, thromboembolism, anemia, bone disease, symptomatic cholelithiasis, chronic fatigue, neurologic abnormalities, depression, food aversion, severe malnutrition and death.

Nutrition, cost and lifestyle are important related considerations. Depending on the patient's choice, nutritional supplementation can cost in the range of $40–$80 per month. Lifestyle is another potential oversight. The management of BPD/DS is time consuming, especially in the early months. Four to six times a day, the patient is required to take supplements and take in nutrition. Until adaptation occurs, bowel movements occur more frequently. Successful patients are proactive in preparing food and planning their supplement schedule. Certain lifestyles and lines of work are not compatible with these rigors.

Preoperative Testing

Preoperative evaluation and preparation in the author's practice include the following: Information session, initial interview, laboratory studies and X-rays, psychiatric evaluation, nutritional consultation, physical therapy consultation, exercise program, consultation with surgeon, PCP-diet program, non-operative weight loss, insurance approval, cardiology consultation, pulmonary consultation, preoperative upper endoscopy, possible preoperative IVC filter, preoperative nutrition classes and mandatory support group.

Postoperative Management

A program with strong follow-up after BPD/DS will achieve the greatest success with fewer nutritional issues in BPD/DS patients. In our experience, the first 18 months postoperatively are the most critical to make adjustments and avoid nutritional deficiencies that would otherwise result in serious clinical consequences. Postoperative visits occur at an increased frequency in the first 18 months. At the least, visits should be scheduled at the following intervals: 1 week, 2 weeks, 1 month, 3 months, 6 months, 1 year, 18 months and then annually for life.

Laboratory testing includes all of the following: Complete blood count, basic metabolic panel, iron studies, calcium, ferritin, folate, intact PTH, prealbumin, total protein, albumin, fasting blood sugar, liver function tests, lipid panel, vitamin B12, zinc, magnesium, vitamin D, vitamin A, vitamin E and thiamine. Testing should be performed at an interval of every 6 months for the first 2 years then annually if there are no abnormalities.

Operative Technique

The procedure can be broken down into four parts: The gastric sleeve, the duodenal dissection, entero-enterostomy and duodeno-ileostomy.

Gastric sleeve

The gastric sleeve is not any different in BPD/DS with the exception that the restrictive component should be less restrictive than a primary vertical sleeve. Careful attention to not encroaching on the incisura, avoiding the gastroesophageal junction and equal capture of tissue anteriorly and posteriorly are paramount.

Duodenal dissection

The duodenal dissection poses the greatest concern regarding possible complications from technical difficulties because of the proximity of the duodenum, common bile duct, portal vein, hepatic artery, pancreas and vena cava. The goal is to transect the duodenum approximately 2–4 cm distal to the pylorus. The lateral dissection starts with a limited exposure of the duodenum at the level of the common bile duct. The medial dissection is retroduodenal and should be kept close to the duodenum and away from the pancreas. After isolation and transection, the proximal duodenum requires further mobilization to create a tension-free anastomosis. Potential problems include adhesions from previous gallbladder surgery and inflammatory adhesions formed from bouts of pancreatitis that may have been subclinical. Injury to the duodenum is always a concern and occurs more frequently in patients with adhesions, especially those in whom the duodenum is adherent to the retroperitoneum and pancreas as a result of previous inflammation. Injury can be treated with primary repair often without great difficulty. Isolating the duodenum first should be considered to determine the feasibility of completing the procedure with a reasonable expectation that the anastomosis can be accomplished.

Entero-enterostomy

The entero-enterostomy is not different than any other small bowel anastomosis. It is important, however, to determine the ability to reach the duodenum before transection. One may consider dividing the omentum, mobilizing the hepatic flexure, or choosing a retrocolic route for the newly created alimentary limb, though none of these are routinely necessary. A separate concern regarding small bowel manipulation is the correct identification and orientation of the limbs at all times. One can easily confuse these components and result in creating blind loops that manifest themselves postoperatively long after leaving the operating room.

Duodeno-ileostomy

As with any other small bowel anastomosis, the approach to this anastomosis can be hand sewn, robotically assisted, or stapled. This author prefers to hand sew the anastomosis because there is little room for error with a stapler when used 2–4 cm from the pylorus. Once a error has occurred after stapling, the only solution may result in a Scopinaro BPD. In this author's view, sutures can be removed with relative ease. Conditions and circumstances that could prove to be prohibitive to performing duodeno-ileostomy include inflammation, active pancreatitis, adherent duodenum, small bowel adhesions preventing mobilization for anastomosis, bleeding and central obesity prohibiting tension-free mobilization of the small bowel.

Early and Late Complications of DS

Overall, the mortality rate and major complications compared to gastric bypass are equal or better in experienced hands.[29,30] Operative mortality has been reported to be 0.1%–1.1%; 90-day mortality is 1.3%.[5,31] DVT and PE rates are 2.2% and 1.1%, respectively. Prolonged operative time and length of stay have been identified as risk factors.[32] Anastomotic leak is a feared early complication that carries a high associated morbidity and mortality. Any suture or staple line is at risk and is greatly influenced by tissue tension, although technical error can also contribute. Small subclinical leaks in stable patients can typically be managed with strict bowel rest, parenteral nutrition, antibiotics and drains; however, an unstable patient requires a return to the operating room. Bowel obstruction can also occur due to internal herniation or adhesions, though the latter is less common in strictly laparoscopic approaches.

It is generally agreed upon to close the mesenteric defect created by the small bowel anastomosis.

Malnutrition/protein malnutrition

Hypoalbuminemia has been reported to be very low or non-existent in patients whose alimentary limbs have been measured as a percentage of the total bowel length. Other methods of measuring bowel length can lead to variable results.[6,31] Assuming patients and bariatric programs are compliant, vulnerability to protein malnutrition is low and requires revision for malabsorption or diarrhea in only 0.7% of patients.[5] As mentioned above, deficiencies in vitamins, iron, calcium and other important minerals will result in a variety of clinical manifestations that need to be addressed on an individualized basis.

Conclusion

BPD/DS requires a special commitment by the patient and a low threshold for intervention at the first sign of malnutrition sequelae. Compliant patients can enjoy good results, the eradication of NIDDM and low recidivism rates.

References

1. Popkin BM. (2007) The world is fat. *Sci Am* **297**(3): 88–95.
2. Prachand VN, Davee RT, Alverdy JC. (2006) Duodenal switch provides superior weight loss in the super-obese (BMI ≥ 52kg/m^2) compared with gastric bypass. *Ann Surg* **244**(4): 611–619.
3. Søvik TT, Aasheim ET, Taha O. (2011) Weight loss, cardiovascular risk factors, and quality of life after gastric bypass and duodenal switch: A randomized trial. *Ann Intern Med* **155**(5): 281–291.
4. Buchwald H, Estok R, Fahrbach K. (2009) Weight and type 2 diabetes after bariatric surgery: Systematic review and meta-analysis. *Am J Med* **122**(3): 248–256.
5. Marceau P, Biron S, Hould FS. (2007) Duodenal switch: Long-term results. *Obes Surg* **17**(11):1421–1430.

6. Hess DS, Hess DW, Oakley RS. (2005) The biliopancreatic diversion with the duodenal switch: Results beyond 10 years. *Obes Surg* **15**(3): 408–416.

7. Deutsch JA. (1978) The stomach in food satiation and the regulation of appetite. *Prog Neurobiol* **10**(3): 135–153.

8. Patriti A, Facchiano E, Sanna A. (2004) The enteroinsular axis and the recovery from type 2 diabetes after bariatric surgery. *Obes Surg* **14**(6): 840–848.

9. Mingrone G, Castagneto-Gissey L. (2009) Mechanisms of early improvement/resolution of type 2 diabetes after bariatric surgery. *Diabetes Metab* **35**(6 Pt 2): 518–523.

10. Spector D, Shikora S. (2010) Neuro-modulation and bariatric surgery for type 2 diabetes mellitus. *Int J Clin Pract Suppl* (**166**): 53–58.

11. Mendieta Zerón H, Domínguez García MV, Camarillo Romero MD *et al.* (2013) Peripheral pathways in the food-intake control towards the adipose-intestinal missing link. *Int J Endocrinol* 598203.

12. Scopinaro N. (2006) Biliopancreatic diversion: Mechanisms of action and long-term results. *Obes Surg* **16**(6): 683–689.

13. Scopinaro N, Gianetta E, Civalleri D. (1979) Bilio-pancreatic bypass for obesity: II. Initial experience in man. *Br J Surg* **66**(9): 618–620.

14. Scopinaro N, Papadia F, Camerini G. (2008) A comparison of a personal series of biliopancreatic diversion and literature data on gastric bypass help to explain the mechanisms of resolution of type 2 diabetes by the two operations. *Obes Surg* **18**(8): 1035–1038.

15. Scopinaro N, Gianetta E, Adami GF. (1996) Biliopancreatic diversion for obesity at eighteen years. *Surgery* **119**(3): 261–268.

16. Scopinaro N, Marinari G, Camerini G *et al.* (2005) Biliopancreatic diversion for obesity: State of the art; 2004 ABS Consensus Conference. *Sur Obes Relat Dis* **1**(3): 317–328.

17. DeMeester TR, Fuchs KH, Ball CS. (1987) Experimental and clinical results with proximal end-to-end duodenojejunostomy for pathologic duodenogastric reflux. *Ann Surg* **206**(4): 414–426.

18. Hess DS, Hess DW. (1998) Biliopancreatic diversion with a duodenal switch. *Obes Surg* **8**(3): 267–282.

19. Hess DS. (2003) Limb measurements in duodenal switch. *Obes Surg* **13**(6): 966.

20. Whitmore C. (2010) Type 2 diabetes and obesity in adults. *Br J Nurs* **19**(14): 880; 882–886.

21. Yusaf S, Hawken S, Ounpuu S. (2005) INTERHEART Study Investigators. Obesity and the risk of myocardial infarction in 27,000 participants from 52 countries: A case-control study. *Lancet* **366**(9497): 1640–1649.
22. Sjöström L, Narbro K, Sjöström CD. (2007) Effects of bariatric surgery on mortality in Swedish obese subjects. *N Engl J Med* **357**(8): 741–752.
23. Strain GW, Gagner M, Pomp A *et al.* (2009) Comparison of weight loss and body composition changes with four surgical procedures. *Surg Obes Relat Dis* **5**(5): 582–587.
24. Madura JA 2nd, DiBaise JK. (2012) Quick fix or long-term cure? Pros and cons of bariatric surgery. *F1000 Med Rep* **4**: 19.
25. Laurenius A, Taha O, Maleckas A. (2010) Laparoscopic biliopancreatic diversion/duodenal switch or laparoscopic Rou-en-Y gastric bypass for super-obesity-weight loss vs side effects. *Surg Obes Relat Dis* **6**(4): 408–414.
26. Sudan R, Bennett KM, Jacobs DO *et al.* (2012) Multifactorial analysis of the learning curve for robot-assisted laparoscopic biliopancreatic diversion with duodenal switch. *Ann Surg* **255**(5): 940–945.
27. Mechanick JI, Youdim A, Jones DB *et al.* (2013) Clinical practice guidelines for the perioperative nutritional, metabolic, and nonsurgical support of the bariatric surgery patient — 2013 update: Cosponsored by American Association of Clinical Endocrinologists, the Obesity Society, and American Society for Metabolic and Bariatric Surgery. *Surg Obes Relat Dis* **9**(2): 159–191.
28. Schweiger C, Keidar A. (2010) Nutritional deficiencies in bariatric surgery patients: prevention, diagnosis and treatment. *Harefuah* **149**(11): 715–720, 748.
29. Biertho L, Lebel S, Marceau S. (2013) Perioperative complications in a consecutive series of 1000 duodenal switches. *Surg Obes Relat Dis* **9**(1): 63–68.
30. Søvik TT, Taha O, Aasheim ET. (2010) Randomized clinical trial of laparoscopic gastric bypass vs laparoscopic duodenal switch for super-obesity. *Br J Surg* **97**(2): 160–166.
31. Keshishian A, Zahriya A, Haroutunian T. (2003) Percentage based bypass of the small intestine results in exceptionally low protein malnutrition. *20th Annual Meeting of the ASBS.*
32. Rezvani M, Sucandy I, Das R *et al.* (2014) Venous thromboembolism after laparoscopic biliopancreatic diversion with duodenal switch: Analysis of 362 patients. *Surg Obes Relat Dis* **10**(3): 469–473.

Chapter 5

Sleeve Gastrectomy: Indications, Procedure and Outcomes

Yalini Vigneswaran* and Michael B. Ujiki*,†

*Northshore University Health System,
2650 RidgeAvenue, Evanston, Illinois, USA
†mujiki@northshore.org

Introduction

Sleeve gastrectomy (SG), also known as a vertical gastrectomy, longitudinal gastrectomy or greater curvature gastrectomy, is a purely restrictive procedure removing approximately 80% of the stomach and leaving a gastric tube about 150cc along the lesser curve. This procedure results in weight loss by two mechanisms: Firstly, by physically reducing the size of the stomach and altering gastric motility, and secondly by decreasing the production of appetite-stimulating hormone, Ghrelin.

Similar to other restrictive bariatric procedures such as gastric banding or gastric bypass, weight loss results from reduced food intake due to the altered capacity of the stomach. However, unlike other restrictive procedures, SG allows for normal eating behavior due to the conservation of stomach anatomy. Although thought of as a purely restrictive procedure, we now understand that Ghrelin,

---

†Corresponding author.

an acylated peptide primarily produced by enteroendocrine cells found in the fundus, is also fundamental to the mechanism of weight loss after SG.[1,2]

In 1988, Hess first developed SG as a modification of biliopancreatic diversion (BPD) and was additionally incorporated with duodenal switch (DS) as part of a complex restrictive and malabsorptive procedure described by Marceau in 1993.[3] It was not until 2000 when the SG was performed as an isolated procedure. When higher morbidity and mortality was observed with super-super obese patients and males in BPD–DS, Gagner's group proposed this restrictive portion of the DS as a first stage procedure in these high-risk patients.[4,5] As this two-stage procedure gained popularity not only for BPD–DS but also roux-en-Y gastric bypass (RYGB),[6] the extent of successful weight loss following the first stage procedure became more evident. Thus due to the clear benefits with low complication rates and simplicity of the procedure, the use of SG as a definite and primary weight loss treatment has grown.[7]

Indications

With the successful results of weight loss and use of this procedure as a primary treatment for obesity, the indications for this operation also continue to grow. Due to the initial controversy surrounding the use of SG, the International Consensus Summit for SG (ICSSG) in 2007 established accepted indications for the procedure as listed in Table 1.[8] As it was historically developed, SG should be considered a first stage of a two-stage procedure (RYGB or BPD–DS) in super-super obese patients (body mass Index [BMI] > 60 kg/m^2). SG is indicated as a primary treatment or as a first stage in super-obese patients, BMI > 50 kg/m^2. Due to the low complication rate as compared to other bariatric procedures, SG is an acceptable primary treatment in patients with a BMI > 40 kg/m^2 with comorbidities that increase the risk for surgery. Patients who cannot undergo a malabsorptive procedure (e.g. Crohn's disease) are appropriate candidates for this purely restrictive procedure. SG is a preferred treatment in those patients that require endoscopic gastric surveillance for any

Table 1 Indications for SG.

Definite SG	Super obese (BMI > 50 kg/m^2).
	High risk obese, super obese or super-super obese.
	History of Crohn's Disease.
	Requiring endoscopic gastric surveillance.
First Stage SG	Super-super obese (BMI > 60 kg/m^2).
	Super obese (BMI > 50 kg/m^2).
	Requiring preoperative weight loss for non-bariatric procedure (orthopedic, transplant).

reason. Lastly, SG can be offered as a first step when another non-bariatric operation requires preoperative weight loss.[9]

Preoperative work up is similar to other bariatric procedures including basic chemistry, complete blood count, thyroid function tests, serum and urine cortisol, serum cholesterol, serum triglycerides and vitamin panel. Additionally all patients undergo psychiatric evaluation and endocrinology work up to rule out any other pathology for metabolic syndrome. Lastly, all patients undergo anesthesia and cardiovascular evaluation prior to surgery.

Procedure

Incision and Exposure: As in all bariatric procedures, trocar placement is crucial. The 15 mm optical port is placed midline 5 to 6 cm inferior to the xiphoid process. The patient is positioned in reverse Trendelenburg to allow for better exposure of the upper abdomen. Under direct vision the two 5 mm working ports are placed at the right and left costal margins. One 5 mm retracting port is placed subxiphoid and the left lateral edge of the liver is retracted cephalad and laterally. A second 5 mm retracting port is placed at the lateral edge of the left rectus to provide downward and lateral traction on the stomach.

Gastrolysis: With retraction of the liver the gastroesophageal junction is exposed and the cardia and angle of Hisare dissected free. The hiatus should be interrogated anteriorly and posteriorly to identify if hiatal herniation is present. When present, a hiatal hernia should always be repaired at the time of the operation. In order to preserve innervation of the pylorus, the vertical division of Latarjet's nerve is spared. The terminal branches of the nerve on the lesser curvature (the Crow's feet) are directly across the greater curvature approximately 6 cm proximal to the pylorus. Thus the pylorus is identified by palpation and the lesser sac is entered 6 cm proximally to allow exposure for resection. The greater omentum is then divided at this point continuing proximally to the angle of His, while remaining close to the stomach and avoiding injury to the spleen. The omentum and the short gastric vessels are carefully divided with the use of a bipolar device.

Gastric Resection: The 60 mm stapling device (4.8 mm staples) is inserted through the 15 mm trocar. With the stomach retracted laterally the stomach is initially divided approximately 2 cm lateral from the lesser curvature. This positioning is intentional to maintain sufficient blood supply and an adequate lumen. At this point a bougie is positioned along the lesser curvature of the stomach beyond the pylorus into the duodenum. On a recent survey at the 4th ICSSG most surgeons chose 36 F blunt-tipped bougie, but surgeon choice ranged from 32–50 F.[10]

The gastrectomy is completed with continuous firings (4.8 mm or 3.5 mm staples) along the bougie up to the angle of His, leaving a gastric pouch as seen in Fig. 1. When completing the resection at the angle of His, the surgeon should remain lateral to fat pad to prevent ischemia of the intra-abdominal esophagus. With completion of the resection, the staple line is inspected for any signs of bleeding or leak. If buttressing is not used for the staple line, an absorbable running suture of the staple line can be performed at the discretion of the surgeon in an attempt to prevent bleeding or leak.

Extraction and Closure: The specimen is removed using an extraction bag through the 15 mm optical port. The bougie is replaced with an endoscope to inspect the staple line. A leak test is performed with the staple line submerged in irrigation and the sleeve is

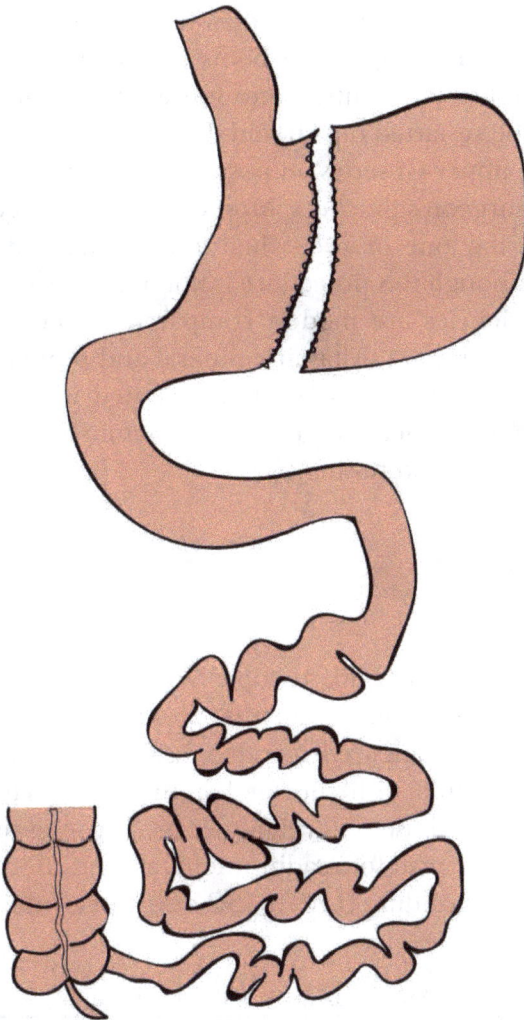

Figure 1.   The remaining gastric tube after the gastric resection is completed.

insufflated. Irrigation is removed, hemostasis is obtained and the trocar sites are closed in standard fashion.

Postoperative Care. All patients are admitted to the monitored floor if no serious medical conditions requiring intensive care monitoring exist. Patients with obstructive sleep apnea are restarted on

home continuous positive airway pressure. All patients are continued on sequential compressive boots and deep vein thrombosis
prophylaxis unless any contraindication exists for anticoagulation.
Patients may be restarted on a liquid diet as seen fit by the surgeon.
Water-soluble upper GI series on postoperative day one may be routine in some surgeon's practices. Most centers discharge patients on
postoperative day one or two, when ambulating and tolerating a
liquid diet. Although this procedure is not malabsorptive and micronutrient deficiencies are modest compared to other procedures,
patients still require multivitamin, mineral and protein supplementation.[11] All patients should be supplemented with multivitamins
and calcium and supplemented for iron, vitamin B12 and vitamin D
based on regular blood testing.[12]

Benefits/Risks

Benefits

As previously eluded to, laparoscopic SG is a preferred procedure
for several reasons (Table 2). First laparoscopic SG is a much simpler procedure as compared to other bariatric operations and in
most cases associated with shorter length of stay. The procedure
does not require the use of foreign objects, negating the associated
complications and need for readjustments as seen after laparoscopic
adjustable gastric banding (LAGB). SG does not create a mesenteric

Table 2   Benefits and risks of SG.

Benefits	Risks
Simple procedure	Staple line bleed/leak
Shorter LOS	Sleeve stricture
No foreign objects	Sleeve dilatation
Anatomy conserved	Weight regain
No mesenteric defect	
No anastomosis/no risk of leak	
Ability to convert to RYGB or BPD–DS	

defect and thus there is no risk for internal hernia. Due to maintenance of the duodenum, pylorus, antrum, lesser curvature and vagal nerve, these patients often continue normal eating behavior and additionally, the anatomy is not significantly altered allowing for access of an endoscope. Since SG does not require an anastomosis, devastating complications of anastomotic leak or stricture do not occur. And lastly, if the desired weight-loss outcome is not observed the procedure can be converted to RYGB or BPD–DS with the completion of the second stage.

Risks

Due to the simplicity of this operation, when compared to other bariatric operations it has a low risk profile, however every procedure has risks. Although there is no anastomosis, the staple line is still at risk for bleeding and/or leak. Peri-operative and postoperative bleeding has been reported to occur at a rate of 1.0%–1.6% of SG cases.[8,13] In fact, the December 2010 ICSSG agreed the staple line should be reinforced to reduce bleeding either by oversewing, applying fibrin sealant or the incorporation of buttressing. Long-term risks include risk of sleeve stricture and the risk of sleeve dilation and weight regain. As in other bariatric surgeries there is always the risk of injuring surrounding structures, such as the liver and spleen.

Outcomes

As surgeons anecdotally saw the significant weight loss after SG as a first step procedure, many started to study patient outcomes after SG alone. In 2006, Himpens *et al.* conducted a randomized control trial comparing restrictive procedures. They showed after randomizing patients to either laparoscopic SG or LAGB, there was significantly better weight loss at three years with SG over LAGB.[1] More recently, Himpens showed that although patients had an average excess weight loss (EWL) of 72.8% at three years, at six year follow-up the mean EWL fell to 57.3%. Of these patients that went on to second-stage

DS, their EWL was 70.8% at six year follow-up.[14] Recently Eid *et al.* demonstrated their long-term outcomes in patients with high BMI. At an average BMI of 66, the eight year follow-up demonstrated an average EWL of 46%.[15]

In addition to weight loss, most bariatric procedures result in remission of obesity-related comorbidities such as diabetes mellitus (DM), gastroesophageal reflux disease (GERD), sleep apnea, hyperlipidemia and hypertension. In a systematic review of 28 studies, 66.2% of patients with DM experienced remission (n = 673).[16] However, it now appears to be unclear whether the type of surgery is a predictor for successful remission. Lee *et al.* randomized gastric bypass vs LSG demonstrated gastric bypass was more effective at resolution of diabetes. However, with a multivariate analysis, the most important predictor of remission was the patient's preoperative duration of diabetes rather than operation.[17]

When Eid *et al.* observed the incidence of GERD in their patients, they saw a biphasic incidence. The symptoms seen at one year follow-up disappeared and were explained by the lack of elasticity, but at six year follow-up, 24% of patients had significant GERD requiring acid suppression therapy. This incidence of GERD was explained by the over eating and stasis of food in the esophagus they saw in these patients.[14] Bohdjalian *et al.* demonstrated similar results after SG with mean EWL at 5 years of 55% at which time 31% of patients required chronic acid suppression.[18] However, the incidence of GERD in these patients remains controversial. A review by Chiu *et al.* showed that most studies did not have an increased incidence of GERD after SG.[19] In fact, Tai *et al.* demonstrated that GERD and erosive gastritis in these patients postoperative was related to the presence of a hiatal hernia, thus emphasizing the importance of repairing hiatal hernias in these patients.[20] Other groups have demonstrated that the incidence of GERD was significantly decreased when hiatal hernia was found and repaired at the time of LSG.[21,22]

When identifying remission of other comorbidities compared to laparoscopic RYGB, SG seems to be comparable. Recently, a randomized prospective trial demonstrated similar outcomes of remission at one year follow-up for sleep apnea, hyperlipidemia, hypertension, diabetes and musculoskeletal disease. The only significant finding was a higher resolution of GERD after RYGB.[23] These results are similar to other retrospective studies comparing SG to RYGB.[24]

Reasons for Failure

Failure of weight loss after the procedure can be due to several reasons. Usually this is associated with dilation of the gastric remnant. This may be due to surgical technique including excessive large bougie and remnant sleeve or inadequate resection of posterior gastric folds. Failure may also occur due to gastric dilation over time and excessive pressure on pouch with large meals or repeated vomiting. Few groups have investigated reoperation and repeating SG for pouch dilation with success. Long-term outcomes for repeating SG needs to be further investigated. However, with failure of SG, patients can experience successful outcomes with conversion to RYGB or BPD–DS.

Conclusion

Although, initially developed as part of a complex bariatric procedure, SG has actually become a popular primary treatment for bariatric surgery. Studies thus far have demonstrated that SG has the potential to be an effective bariatric procedure for weight loss and remission of comorbidities in the bariatric population with minimal complications. Additionally SG also allows for revision and conversion to a more complex bariatric operation if weight loss is not achieved. We believe SG is a simple and efficacious bariatric procedure that should be among the choices when surgeons discuss bariatric procedures with patients, in particular high-risk patients.

References

1. Himpens J, Dapri G, Cadière GB. (2006) A prospective randomized study between laparoscopic gastric banding and laparoscopic isolated

sleeve gastrectomy: Results after 1 and 3 years. *Obes Surg* **16**(11): 1450–1456.

2. Mognol P, Chosidow D, Marmuse JP. (2005) Laparoscopic sleeve gastrectomy as an initial bariatric operation for high-risk patients: Initial results in 10 patients. *Obes Surg* **15**(7): 1030–1033.

3. Hess DS, Hess DW. (1998) Biliopancreatic diversion with a duodenal switch. *Obes Surg* **8**(3): 267–282.

4. Fazylov RM, Savel RH, Horovitz JH, Pagala MK, Coppa GF, Nicastro J, Lazzaro RS, Macura JM. (2005) Association of super-super-obesity and male gender with elevated mortality in patients undergoing the duodenal switch procedure. *Obes Surg* **15**(5): 618–623.

5. Ren CJ, Patterson E, Gagner M. (2000) Early results of laparoscopic biliopancreatic diversion with duodenal switch: A case series of 40 consecutive patients. *Obes Surg* **10**(6): 514–523; discussion 524.

6. Regan JP, Inabnet WB, Gagner M, Pomp A. (2003) Early experience with two-stage laparoscopic Roux-en-Y gastric bypass as an alternative in the super-super obese patient. *Obes Surg* **13**(6): 861–864.

7. Cottam D, Qureshi FG, Mattar SG Sharma S, Holover S, Bonanomi G, Ramanathan R, Schauer P. (2006) Laparoscopic sleeve gastrectomy as an initial weight-loss procedure for high-risk patients with morbid obesity. *Surg Endosc* **20**(6): 859–863.

8. Deitel M, Crosby RD, Gagner M. (2008) The first international consensus summit for sleeve gastrectomy (SG), New York City, October 25–27, 2007. *Obes Surg* **18**(5): 487–496.

9. Tucker ON, Szomstein S, Rosenthal RJ. (2008) Indications for sleeve gastrectomy as a primary procedure for weight loss in the morbidly obese. *J Gastrointest Surg* **12**(4): 662–667.

10. Gagner M, Deitel M, Erickson AL, Crosby RD. (2013) Survey on laparoscopic sleeve gastrectomy (LSG) at the fourth international consensus summit on sleeve gastrectomy. *Obes Surg* **23**(12): 2013–2017.

11. Damms-Machado A, Friedrich A, Kramer KM, Stingel K, Meile T, Küper MA, Königsrainer A, Bischoff SC. (2012) Pre- and postoperative nutritional deficiencies in obese patients undergoing laparoscopic sleeve gastrectomy. *Obes Surg* **22**(6): 881–889.

12. Aarts EO, Janssen IM, Berends FJ. (2011) The gastric sleeve: Losing weight as fast as micronutrients? *Obes Surg* **21**(2): 207–211.

13. Gagner M, Deitel M, Kalberer TL, Erickson AL, Crosby RD. (2009) The second international consensus summit for sleeve gastrectomy, March 19–21, 2009. *Surg Obes Relat Dis* **5**(4): 476–485.

14. Himpens J, Dobbeleir J, Peeters G. (2010) Long-term results of laparoscopic sleeve gastrectomy for obesity. *Ann Surg* **252**(2): 319–324.

15. Eid GM, Brethauer S, Mattar SG, Titchner RL, Gourash W, Schauer PR. (2012) Laparoscopic sleeve gastrectomy for super obese patients: Forty-eight percent excess weight loss after 6 to 8 years with 93% follow-up. *Ann Surg* **256**(2): 262–265.

16. Gill RS, Birch DW, Shi X, Sharma AM, Karmali S. (2010) Sleeve gastrectomy and type 2 diabetes mellitus: A systematic review. *Surg Obes Relat Dis* **6**(6): 707–713.

17. Lee WJ, Chong K, Ser KH, Lee YC, Chen SC, Chen JC, Tsai MH, Chuang LM. (2011) Gastric bypass vs sleeve gastrectomy for type 2 diabetes mellitus: A randomized controlled trial. *Arch Surg* **146**(2): 143–148.

18. Bohdjalian A, Langer FB, Shakeri-Leidenmühler S, Gfrerer L, Ludvik B, Zacherl J, Prager G. (2010) Sleeve gastrectomy as sole and definitive bariatric procedure: 5-year results for weight loss and ghrelin. *Obes Surg* **20**(5): 535–540.

19. Chiu S, Birch DW, Shi X, Sharma AM, KarmaliS. (2011) Effect of sleeve gastrectomy on gastroesophageal reflux disease: A systematic review. *Surg Obes Relat Dis* **7**(4): 510–515.

20. Tai CM, Huang CK. (2013) Increase in gastroesophageal reflux disease symptoms and erosive esophagitis 1 year after laparoscopic sleeve gastrectomy among obese adults. *Surg Endosc* **27**(10): 3937.

21. Soricelli E, Iossa A, Casella G, Abbatini F, Calì B, Basso N. (2013) Sleeve gastrectomy and crural repair in obese patients with gastroesophageal reflux disease and/or hiatal hernia. *Surg Obes Relat Dis* **9**(3): 356–361.

22. Daes J, Jimenez ME, Said N, Daza JC, Dennis R. (2012) Laparoscopic sleeve gastrectomy: Symptoms of gastroesophageal reflux can be reduced by changes in surgical technique. *Obes Surg* **22**(12): 1874–1879.

23. Peterli R, Borbély Y, Kern B, Gass M, Peters T, Thurnheer M, Schultes B, Laederach K, Bueter M, Schiesser M. (2013) Early results of the Swiss multicentre bypass or sleeve study (SM-BOSS): A prospective randomized trial comparing laparoscopic sleeve gastrectomy and Roux-en-Y gastric bypass. *Ann Surg* **258**(5): 690–694; discussion 695.

24. Vidal P, Ramón JM, Goday A, Benaiges D, Trillo L, Parri A, González S, Pera M, Grande L. (2013) Laparoscopic gastric bypass vs laparoscopic sleeve gastrectomy as a definitive surgical procedure for morbid obesity. Mid-term results. *Obes Surg* **23**(3): 292–299.

Chapter 6

Comparative Outcomes in Bariatric Surgery

Christopher R. Daigle and Stacy A. Brethauer*

Bariatric and Metabolic Institute
Cleveland Clinic, Cleveland, OH, USA
*brethas@ccf.org

Introduction

Generating high quality studies comparing the safety, efficacy and outcomes of surgical procedures can be challenging given the numerous methodological and ethical issues that surround procedural-based scientific endeavors. Much of the scientific literature that exists pertaining to surgery is retrospective in nature or examines prospective cohorts without randomized comparison groups. Randomized control trials (RCTs) are widely accepted as the gold standard methodological approach to compare multiple medical therapies, surgical vs medical treatment or different surgical approaches. Unfortunately, well-designed RCTs make up a minority of the body of surgical literature due to a myriad of issues including the timing of surgical trials, issues with standardization of procedures, difficulties in blinding of subjects and investigators, ethical issues specific to surgical trials and concern surrounding clinical equipoise.[1,2]

---

*Corresponding author.

Bariatric and metabolic surgery has become one of the most studied fields in medicine, with an ever-growing abundance of new studies surfacing every year. Many systematic reviews, meta-analyses and RCTs have now been published that offer significant (and often comparative) data that can aid clinicians and patients in making informed decisions with regards to procedural approach, balancing of risks and benefits and the metabolic benefits of bariatric surgery. This chapter aims to highlight some of the major landmark comparative studies that have helped shape bariatric and metabolic surgery into the contemporary field it is today.

Comparative Outcomes of Bariatric Surgical Approaches

In 2004, Buchwald *et al.* published their systematic review and meta-analysis of bariatric surgery outcomes, a study that has become one of the most cited papers in bariatric and metabolic surgery.[3,4] The systematic analysis extracted 136 studies with 91 overlapping populations for a total of 22,094 bariatric surgical patients. The total cohort was comprised of 72.6% females and 19.4% males, with a mean age of 39 years and a baseline mean BMI of 46.9 (range, 32.3–68.8). Using a random effects model, Buchwald was able to assess the efficacy (expressed as excess weight loss (EWL)) and mortality of the various bariatric surgical procedures. The operative mortality rates, defined as mortality within 30 days of the operation, were 0.1% for purely restrictive procedures (gastroplasty, banding), 0.5% for those who had gastric bypass and 1.1% for subjects who had biliopancreatic diversion or duodenal switch. The mean EWL for the entire meta-analysis cohort in Buchwald's study was 61.2% (61.5%–74.8%). The most efficacious procedure in the cohort was biliopancreatic diversion or duodenal switch with an EWL of 70.1% (66.3%–73.9%), followed by gastroplasty (mainly VBG) (68.2%, 61.5%–74.8%), gastric bypass (61.6%, 56.7%–66.5%) and gastric banding (adjustable and non-adjustable) (47.5%, 40.7%–54.2%). The study also assessed the metabolic effects of the various weight loss procedures by assessing remission or improvement of obesity-related comorbidities such as diabetes mellitus, hyperlipidemia, hypertension and obstructive sleep apnea (OSA). Diabetes was completely resolved in 76.8% of patients undergoing a bariatric procedure, with improvement seen in 86.0% of the meta-cohort. There was also a difference in diabetes resolution seen between the 4 types of procedures: 98.9% (95% CI, 96.8%–100%) for biliopancreatic diversion or duodenal switch, 83.7% (95% CI, 77.3%–90.1%) for gastric bypass, 71.6% (95% CI, 55.1%–88.2%) for gastroplasty and 47.9% (95% CI, 29.1%–66.7%) for gastric banding. The maximum improvement in hyperlipidemia was observed in the biliopancreatic or duodenal switch (99.1%, 95% CI, 97.6%–100%) and the gastric bypass (96.9%, 95% CI, 93.6%–100%) groups. Hypertension resolved in 61.7% of the cohort, with improvement in 78.5%, but the rank order of the various procedures with respect to hypertension was variable. The total percentage of patients who experienced resolution of OSA in the meta-analysis was 85.7%.[3]

In 2011, Nguyen *et al.* published the first report from the American College of Surgeons Bariatric Surgery Center Network (ACS-BSCN), a study that ultimately placed laparoscopic sleeve gastrectomy (LSG) in between banding and gastric bypass with respect to morbidity and effectiveness. The ACS-BSCN accreditation program was a prospective and longitudinal database that captured multi-institutional, nationwide data on bariatric surgery cases and it was used in this study to compare sleeve gastrectomy to gastric banding and gastric bypass. In total, 28,616 patients from 109 hospitals were included and various outcomes were assessed; 944 cases were LSG, 12,193 were laparoscopic adjustable gastric bands (LAGB), 14,491 were laparoscopic Roux-en-Y gastric bypass (RYGB) and 988 were open RYGB. The conclusion of this study was that LSG has a morbidity and efficacy that falls between LAGB and open or laparoscopic RYGB. Specifically, they found that LSG had a statistically significant higher 30-day morbidity (5.61% vs 1.44%, $p < 0.05$), readmission (5.4% vs 1.17%, $p < 0.05$) and re-operative rate (2.97% vs 0.92%, $p < 0.05$) when compared to banding; however, re-operation and intervention rates were lower for LSG when compared to gastric bypass (re-operation rates for LSG, laparoscopic RYGB and open RYGB were 2.9%, 5.02% and 5.06%, respectively; $p < 0.05$ in both cases). Furthermore, the absolute BMI reduction after LSG was found to be less than the weight loss achieved by open or laparoscopic gastric bypass, but greater than that seen with LAGB at 6 months and 1 year follow-up. When they assessed the effectiveness of the 3 bariatric procedures on obesity-related comorbidities (diabetes, hypertension, hyperlipidemia, OSA), they also found the same trend: LSG was positioned between banding and bypass. Of note, LSG was found to be less effective than the other two operations at improving GERD.[5]

The Michigan Bariatric Surgery Collective recently released their prospective, externally audited, statewide data aimed at clarifying the effectiveness, morbidity and mortality of LSG when compared to LAGB and laparoscopic RYGB. The study matched 2949 LSG patients to equal numbers of RYGB and LAGB subjects for 23 baseline parameters and looked at various outcomes for up to 3 years postoperatively. The overall 30-day complication rate was 6.3% for LSG, which was significantly higher than LAGB (2.4%, $p < 0.0001$), but lower than RYGB (10.0%, $p < 0.0001$). When adjusting for serious complications only, LSG had a similar rate to RYGB (2.4% vs 2.5%, $p = 0.736$), which was higher than for LAGB (1.0%, $p < 0.0001$). There was no significant difference in mortality rates for the 3 groups (0.10 for RYGB, 0.07 for LSG and 0.07 for LAGB). At 1-year follow-up, the mean EWL for the LSG cohort was 60.0%, which was significantly lower than for RYGB (69%, $p < 0.0001$), but considerably higher than for LAGB (34%, $p < 0.0001$). As for obesity-related comorbidity outcomes, LSG also appeared to have an effect closer to RYGB than LAGB. They reported non-insulin-dependent diabetes remission in 80% of RYGB patients, 66% in LSG and 37% in LAGB. The study also looked at insulin dependent diabetics and found remission in 64% of RYGB subjects, 42% of LSG patients and 32% in those who underwent LAGB. When compared to LAGB and RYGB, LSG had statistically higher diabetes remission (both insulin and non-insulin dependent) rates than LAGB, but had lower rates when compared to RYGB ($p < 0.05$ for both comparisons). Other comorbid conditions assessed included hypertension (45% resolution in RYGB, 40% LSG, 18% LAGB), hyperlipidemia (63% remission in RYGB, 40% LSG, 27% LAGB) and sleep apnea (66% remission in RYGB, 57% LSG, 29% LAGB). The authors concluded that LSG has a superior safety profile to RYGB and has outcomes that are superior to LAGB.[6]

Surgery vs Medical Therapy for the Treatment of Type 2 Diabetes

There have been numerous RCTs that have demonstrated the ability of bariatric surgery to provide more effective and durable therapy for morbid obesity and obesity-related comorbidities than medical therapy alone. These trials helped change the focus of bariatric surgery from weight loss outcomes to metabolic outcomes.

A randomized study by O'Brien *et al.* addressed the efficacy of LAGB compared to intensive medical therapy for the treatment of mild-to-moderate obesity (BMI of 30–35) in 80 patients.[7] Intensive medical treatment consisted of 24 months of very low calorie diets, lifestyle modification and pharmacotherapy. At 2 years, the surgical group had greater EWL than the medical therapy group (87.2% vs 21.8%, $p < 0.002$) and also scored significantly higher on subjective quality of life assessments. The trial also assessed the effects of both therapeutic approaches on metabolic syndrome, which was defined based on the ATP III criteria. [8] At the onset of the study, 15 patients (38%) in each group met the ATP III criteria for metabolic syndrome. At 2 years follow-up, 8 (24%) of the non-surgical patients and 1 (3%) of the surgical patients still had metabolic syndrome ($p < 0.002$).[7]

In O'Brien's RCTs, they reported adverse events in 18 (58%) non-surgical patients and 7 (18%) of the surgical arm, with no mortalities in either arm. However, it should be noted that the majority of "adverse events" in the medical arm were intolerance to the prescribed diets ($n = 9$) and loss to follow-up ($n = 5$). The surgical arm did require 5 (13%) operative interventions for 4 (10%) slipped bands and one episode of acute cholecystitis. The study concluded that surgical treatment using LAGB was statistically significantly more effective than intensive medical therapy at reducing weight, improving quality of life and treating metabolic syndrome.[7] As previously mentioned, LAGB has been shown to be less effective at weight reduction than procedures like LSG and RYGB and the findings of this study sparked considerable interest in exploring the effect these more efficacious procedures could have on metabolic diseases, like diabetes mellitus.

In 2012, two separate RCTs were simultaneously published comparing bariatric surgery to conventional or intensive medical therapy for type 2 diabetes.[9,10] Previous studies had identified a link between bariatric surgery and improvement or remission of type 2 diabetes, but these trials were the first well-designed randomized control studies assessing this effect. Mingrone and colleagues' study was a single-center, randomized, non-blinded, controlled trial that included 60 patients aged 30–60 years with a BMI of 35 or more and a diagnosis of diabetes for at least 5 years duration. Patients were randomized to 1 of 3 arms: 20 patients were assigned to biliopancreatic diversion, 20 patients to gastric bypass and 20 patients to conventional medical therapy for diabetes. Their primary end point was the rate of diabetes remission at 2-year follow-up, defined as a fasting glucose level <100 mg and a glycated hemoglobin (HbA1c) <6.5%. Their analysis demonstrated that 95% of the biliopancreatic patients and 75% of the gastric bypass patients achieved diabetes remission, whereas none of the medical therapy patients achieved remission ($p < 0.001$ when both surgical arms were compared to medical therapy). All three groups did exhibit reductions in HbA1c at the 2-year end point, but the improvement was more pronounced in the surgical groups (7.69 ± 0.57% for medical therapy, 6.35 ± 1.42% for gastric bypass and 4.95 ± 0.49% for biliopancreatic diversion). Of note, their analysis found that age, sex, baseline BMI, weight changes and diabetes duration were not predictors of diabetes remission or improvement in glucose levels in 1- and 3- month follow-up. The authors concluded that bariatric surgery resulted in better glucose control than medical therapy in morbidly obese diabetic patients.[9]

Schauer *et al.*'s study was also a non-blinded, single-center trial with 150 morbidly obese poorly controlled type 2 diabetic patients randomized at a 1:1:1 ratio to either intensive medical therapy alone, medical therapy plus gastric bypass or medical therapy plus sleeve gastrectomy. The group had a mean age of 49 ± 8 years, 66% were female and the average HbA1c was 9.2 ± 1.5%. Compared to

Mingrone's study, Schauer's RCTs had a more stringent definition of diabetes remission (HbA1c < 6.0%) at a study end point of 12 months follow-up. Their analysis found that 12% (5 of 41) of medical therapy patients achieved their definition of remission vs 42% (21 of 50, $p = 0.002$) in the gastric bypass plus medical therapy group and 37% (18 of 49, $p = 0.008$) in the sleeve gastrectomy plus medical therapy group. Much like Mingrone's trial, this RCT did demonstrate glycemic improvement in all groups, but with a more pronounced effect in the surgical arms. The mean HbA1c at 12 months was $7.5 \pm 1.8\%$ for the medical group, $6.4 \pm 0.9\%$ in the gastric bypass group and $6.6 \pm 1.0\%$ in the sleeve group. Also, the use of lipid reducing agents, anti-hypertensive and glycemic control medications were significantly reduced in the surgical arms, whereas the need for these medications increased in the intensive medical therapy group. The authors concluded that 12 months of bariatric surgery plus medical therapy was superior to intensive medical therapy alone in achieving glycemic control in morbidly obese patients with uncontrolled type 2 diabetes.[10]

Finally, Gloy *et al.* recently published a systematic review and meta-analysis assessing existing RCTs on bariatric surgery vs non-surgical treatment for obesity and the metabolic outcomes achieved. The meta-analysis included 11 studies for a total of 796 individuals with a BMI ranging from 30–52. They found that patients allocated to bariatric surgery had better weight loss (mean difference -26 kg) compared to non-surgical therapy, higher remission rates for type 2 diabetes (relative risk of 22.1), more improvement of metabolic syndrome (relative risk of 2.4), greater improvement in the cohort's quality of life scores and an overall decrease in medications needed for comorbid conditions. With respect to metabolic parameters, the analysis found significantly lower triglyceride and higher HDL cholesterol levels in those who underwent surgical therapy. Of note, there was no significant difference in blood pressure control or LDL cholesterol levels between surgical and non-surgical cohorts.[11]

Conclusion

There are several key studies that have advanced our understanding of the safety and efficacy of the various contemporary bariatric surgical procedures and the effect they have on obesity-related comorbid conditions. High quality research continues worldwide in an attempt to understand the exact mechanisms of comorbid disease resolution. As more comparative data emerges, the long-term risks and benefits of the various bariatric procedures will become clear and this data will assist surgeons in patient and procedural selection.

References

1. McLeod RS. (1999) Issues in surgical randomized controlled trials. *World J Surg* **23**(12): 1210–1214.
2. McDonald PJ, Kulkarni AV, Farrokhyar F *et al.* (2010) Ethical issues in surgical research. *Can J Surg* **53**(2): 133–136.
3. Buchwald H, Avidor Y, Braunwald E *et al.* (2004) Bariatric surgery: A systematic review and meta-analysis. *JAMA* **292**(14): 1724–1737.
4. Aminian A, Daigle CR, Brethauer SA *et al.* (2014) Citation classics: Top 50 cited articles in bariatric and metabolic surgery. *Surg Obes Relat Dis.* In Press, Uncorrected Proof, Available online 29 January 2014. [http://dx.doi.org/10.1016/j.soard.2013.12.021].
5. Hutter MM, Schirmer BD, Jones DB *et al.* (2011) First report from the American College of Surgeons Bariatric Surgery Center Network: Laparoscopic sleeve gastrectomy has morbidity and effectiveness positioned between the band and the bypass. *Ann Surg* **254**(3): 410–420.
6. Carlin AM, Zeni TM, English WJ *et al.* (2013) Michigan Bariatric Surgery Collaborative. The comparative effectiveness of sleeve gastrectomy, gastric bypass, and adjustable gastric banding procedures for the treatment of morbid obesity. *Ann Surg* **257**(5): 791–797.
7. O'Brien PE, Dixon JB, Laurie C *et al.* (2006) Treatment of mild to moderate obesity with laparoscopic adjustable gastric banding or an intensive medical program: A randomized trial. *Ann Intern Med* **144**(9): 625–633.
8. Expert Panel on Detection, Evaluation, and Treatment of High Blood Cholesterol in Adults. (2001) Executive Summary of the Third Report of the National Cholesterol Education Program (NCEP) Expert Panel on Detection, Evaluation, and Treatment of High Blood Cholesterol in Adults (Adult Treatment Panel III). *JAMA* **285**(19): 2486–2497.

9. Mingrone G, Panunzi S, De Gaetano A *et al.* (2012) Bariatric surgery versus conventional medical therapy for type 2 diabetes. *N Engl J Med* **366**(17): 1577–1585.
10. Schauer PR, Kashyap SR, Wolski K *et al.* (2012) Bariatric surgery versus intensive medical therapy in obese patients with diabetes. *N Engl J Med* **366**(17): 1567–1576.
11. Gloy VL, Briel M, Bhatt DL *et al.* (2013) Bariatric surgery versus non-surgical treatment for obesity: A systematic review and meta-analysis of randomised controlled trials. *BMJ* **347**: f5934.

Chapter 7

Complications of Bariatric Surgery and Management

Bill Ran Luo* and Alex Nagle*,†

*Department of Surgery,
Northwestern University, Feinberg School of Medicine
676 N. St. Clair Ave, Suite 6-650 Chicago, IL 60611
†anagle@nmh.org

Introduction

Bariatric surgery has proved to be the most effective treatment of severe obesity and its associated co-morbidities. In 2010, it is estimated that 160,000 bariatric surgeries were performed in the U.S. Given the high surgical volume, improving the safety of these operations has become a high priority, leading to the development of strict criteria for center accreditation, guidelines for safe and effective bariatric surgery, and careful monitoring of surgical outcomes. These efforts have been an important step forward in an attempt to deliver bariatric surgery in a manner as safely as possible. In addition, most surgeons have moved beyond the learning curve for laparoscopic techniques, further improving the safety of laparoscopic bariatric surgery over the past decade. Nonetheless, complications following bariatric surgery remain a significant concern. Complications can be

---

†Corresponding author.

categorized as early (within 30-day postoperative) and late (beyond 30-day postoperative) and vary based upon the specific procedure performed. There are also patient-specific risk factors that will influence morbidity and mortality. Overall, complications occur in about 7.3% of patients, major life-threatening complications in 2.3%, and 30-day mortality rate of 0.1%.[1,2] This chapter will review the major complications of bariatric surgery and discuss their respective management, focusing on the three most commonly performed procedures in the US: Laparoscopic Roux-en-Y gastric bypass (RYGB), laparoscopic adjustable gastric band (LAGB), and laparoscopic sleeve gastrectomy (LSG).

Early Complications

Mortality

The overall 30-day mortality for bariatric surgical procedures is less than 1%. This compares favorably with the hospital mortality of other frequently performed major surgical procedures including hip replacement (0.3%), abdominal aneurysm repair (3.9%), esophageal resection (9.1%) and pancreatic resection (8.3%). The most common causes of early mortality are pulmonary emboli and complications related to leaks. Several factors have been associated with an increased mortality risk. A study of 16,155 Medicare beneficiaries (mean age, 47.7 years) who underwent bariatric procedures reported a 3-fold higher mortality rate for those aged 65 and older compared with younger patients.[2] The same study also reported that male gender is a risk factor for increasing mortality (3.7 vs 1.5% at 30 days, 4.8 vs 2.1% at 90 days and 7.5 vs 3.7% at 1 year). Super-obesity (BMI > 50) and chronic disease such as underlying pulmonary and cardiac disease contribute to an increased risk of death with bariatric surgical procedures. Increased mortality is also associated with low surgeon and hospital volume of bariatric procedures. Both in-hospital and 30-day mortality are decreased when bariatric surgery is performed by surgeons and hospitals that perform more than 100 procedures a year. For these reasons, volume is one of the criteria utilized by the American Society for Metabolic and Bariatric Surgery (ASMBS) and the American College of Surgeons for the accreditation of bariatric center of excellence programs.

Risk assessment and stratification is important in the decision to perform weight loss surgery. A scoring system to predict mortality in gastric bypass patients has been derived and then validated in a separate population. Using body mass index (BMI), male gender, hypertension, pulmonary embolus risk and age, patients were grouped into three risk categories: Low (Class A), intermediate (Class B) and high (Class C). The differences in mortality rates among the three risk classes was significant; Class A, 0.3%, Class B, 1.9% and Class C, 7.6%.

Readmission and reoperation

Complications from bariatric procedures may lead to the need for re-hospitalization and reoperation. Given the large numbers of bariatric procedures performed, re-hospitalizations and reoperations for bariatric surgery represent significant costs for hospitals and insurance companies. In a report from ASMBS Centers of Excellence with data from 2005–2007, the readmission rate was 5% and reoperation rate was 2%. In a study of 1939 consecutive bariatric operations at a high volume bariatric center, laparoscopic RYGB had the highest readmission rate of 24% while LAGB had the lowest readmission rate of 13%.[3]

Deep vein thrombosis (DVT) and pulmonary embolism (PE)

PE is the most common cause of 30-day mortality following bariatric surgery and can account for more than 50% of deaths. The incidence of symptomatic DVT ranges from 0%–5.4%, and for PE 0%–6.4%.[4] Optimal strategies for preventing DVT/PE have not been established, but at a minimum, the ASMBS recommends early postoperative ambulation, the use of lower extremity sequential compression devices (SCDs), and chemoprophylaxis with either subcutaneous unfractionated heparin or low-molecular weight

heparin. Preoperative risk stratification is an important tool to identifying high-risk patients which may benefit from more aggressive
prophylaxis. Risk factors associated with fatal PE include severe
venous stasis disease, BMI > 60, truncal obesity, immobility, history of
a prior DVT/PE and obesity-hypoventilation syndrome. In patients
identified preoperatively as high-risk for PE, chemoprophylaxis with
low-molecular weight heparin can be prescribed for an extended
period beyond discharge from the hospital. Some groups also advo-
cate for the selective use of retrievable inferior vena cava (IVC) fil-
ters in high-risk patients, but this is center dependent.[25]

Diagnosis of PE in morbidly obese patients can be problematic
because use of standard diagnostic modalities (nuclear lung scan or
CT-angiography) may be limited and not physically feasible in super
obese patients. Immediate anticoagulation is indicated for patients
for whom there is a high level of clinical suspicion. In patients in
whom anticoagulation is contraindicated, an IVC filter can be utilized to lower the risk of continued clot propagation.

Surgical site infections (SSI)

SSI can occur with any bariatric procedures, with an overall incidence of 2.7%.[1] The American Society of Health-System Pharmacists
currently recommends preoperative intravenous Cefazolin 2 g (3 g
for >120 kg) to be given within 1 h of the skin incision and re-dosing
at 4 h. In LSG, the most commonly infected site is the extraction
port for the resected stomach. There are many techniques for
extraction, such as utilizing a commercially available wound protec-
tors, endoscopic bag devices, or removal without any skin protec-
tion. There does not appear to be any significant correlations in the
extraction technique and subsequent SSI.[5] When utilizing the circular stapler technique in laparoscopic RYGB, the incision site of
greatest concern is where the circular staple is passed through the
abdominal wall. Various strategies have been described to minimize
the risk of SSI at this incision. Signs of a developing SSI in a bariatric
surgery patient should be addressed quickly. Although the morbidity for a patient from having an open wound is a valid concern,

opening the wound will allow for drainage of any potentially infected fluid, protect deeper tissues and prevent wound dehiscence or even evisceration.

Cardiac complications

Although most morbidly obese patients undergo a vigorous clearance process prior to bariatric surgery, cardiac complications such as myocardial infarction or atrial fibrillation are still of concern. Due to the nature of the operations the patient may have epigastric and shoulder pain, which can lead to a missed cardiac ischemic event. Based on the clinician's degree of suspicion an electrocardiogram, cardiac enzymes and appropriate consultation of the cardiology team should be obtained. Despite the concerns, overall cardiac complications for bariatric surgeries are very low, ranging from an incidence of 0.04%–0.14%.[1]

Late Complications

Gallstones

Rapid weight loss can contribute to the development of gallstones by increasing the lithogenicity of bile. RYGB patients are more likely to require cholecystectomy compared to LAGB and LSG patients. A review of 1,715 bariatric surgeries reported that 4.2% of patients required laparoscopic cholecystectomy during follow-up that ranged from 2 weeks and 68 months.[6] The incidence of laparoscopic cholecystectomy was highest during the first six months after bariatric surgery and then declined over time (55.4%, 21.6%, 14.9%, 5.4% and 2.7% at 1, 2, 3, 4 and 5 years follow-up respectively). Almost all patients requiring cholecystectomy present with biliary colic, and very few present with acute cholecystitis. Given the low rate (approximately 5%) of cholecystectomy following bariatric surgery, the common practice in the laparoscopic era has been not to routinely perform cholecystectomy at the time of the bariatric surgery. However, if the patient presents with symptomatic gallstones preoperatively, it is best to remove the gallbladder at the time of bariatric surgery. The surgical opinion about asymptomatic gallstones is more divided, and studies have failed to demonstrate the benefit for simultaneous cholecystectomy for incidental gallstones at the time of RYGB.

Patients can also develop common bile duct stones, which can be difficult to treat in the postoperative RYGB patient. Diagnosis of choledocholithiasis can be confirmed by ultrasound or magnetic resonance cholangiopancreatography (MRCP). Endoscopic intervention and management can be problematic due to the altered anatomy of the Roux-en-Y configuration causing relative inaccessibility to the duodenum. As a result, successful endoscopic retrograde cholangiopancreatography (ERCP) with cannulation of the papilla is very difficult to perform and treatment of choledocholithiasis requires either surgical or transhepatic percutaneous access. If the patient has not had a cholecystectomy, then the initial approach should be a laparoscopic cholecystectomy with intra-operative cholangiogram and laparoscopic trans-cystic common bile duct exploration (CBDE). If laparoscopic CBDE is not feasible, then a laparoscopic-assisted ERCP with direct placement of the ERCP scope via a 15 mm trocar into the gastric remnant has been performed with good results. Alternatively, placement of a gastrostomy tube into the bypassed stomach at the time of gastric bypass, with the addition of a radiopaque marker to facilitate future percutaneous access to the gastric remnant has also been described.

Trocar and incisional hernias

Morbid obesity is associated with increased intra-abdominal pressure and susceptibility to the development of abdominal wall hernias. Fortunately, with the advent of laparoscopy, incisional hernias have been minimized. The reported incidence of trocar site hernia is 0.6%, with a median time to presentation of 8–13 months.[7] Trocar site hernias can be difficult to diagnose after surgery. Any concerning signs of obstruction or worsening pain should prompt imaging studies or exploration.

Repair of most hernias following bariatric surgery should be delayed until the patient has achieved significant weight loss. Typically the hernia repair can be safely performed via a laparoscopic approach. However, if the patient also requires a panniculectomy, an open incisional hernia repair can be performed at the same time.

Procedure Specific Complications

LAGB

Band slippage

Band slippage involves prolapse of part of the stomach through the band, with varying degrees of gastric obstruction. Anterior prolapse involves migration of the band cephalad which creates an acute angle with the stomach pouch and esophagus, resulting in obstruction. Posterior gastric prolapse occurs when the stomach migrates cephalad, displacing the band caudally and creating a new pouch. The incidence of band slippage is dependent on the technique during insertion. The earlier experience with the LAGB placement via the perigastric technique had a slippage rate of 20% compared to the later pars flaccida approach, which reduced slippage rates to 2%.[8] There can be early slippage within the first week postoperatively, but the majority occur on average 12 months postoperatively. A slipped band causes a relative outlet obstruction and the patient typically presents with nausea, emesis and inability to take anything orally. Initial management involves volume resuscitation and removal of all fluid from the subcutaneous port. Diagnostically, an upright abdominal X-ray can be used to see the presence of a slippage. The angle of the spine with the orientation of the band (phi angle) is typically 55 degrees, and the shape of the band is described as rectangular. When slippage has occurred the band takes more of an "O" shape, and the phi angle flattens.[9] Fluoroscopy is typically necessary to confirm the diagnosis of a slipped band and can evaluate the severity of intraluminal obstruction. A CT-scan may add additional information, but is usually unnecessary.

The timing of intervention is dependent on the passage of contrast fluoroscopic studies. If contrast freely flows past the band then there is no need for emergent surgical intervention for removal of the band. A discussion should be held between the bariatric surgeon and the patient regarding the goals of weight loss. If the patient desires continued weight loss, band repositioning can be considered, but patients may be better served with conversion to either a RYGB or LSG. Patients who undergo band removal alone without conversion to another bariatric procedure are at high risk for weight re-gain. However, if contrast does not pass through the area of the band indicating a complete obstruction, then prompt surgical intervention should be pursued with the understanding that future revisional surgery would still be an option.[21]

Band erosion

Band erosion is thought to occur secondary to localized inflammation from the synthetic material next to the gastric wall causing the band to erode through the wall into the lumen. The largest retrospective study to date by Brown *et al.*[10] observed that in 865 patients 88% presented with lack of satiety, and 26% had port site related complications. Abdominal pain was present in about a 5th of the patients. Surprisingly, no patients had symptoms of hematemesis or hemorrhage. In this case series they identified an incidence of 2.85%, but other papers have sited erosion to occur in as high as 30% of patients. Endoscopy is usually diagnostic and can be used in combination with an intra-abdominal approach for therapeutic intervention. Excision and removal of the band, with repair of the defect in the stomach is curative. Depending on the patient's wishes and weight loss results a new band can be placed, but Brown's data shows that the rates of re-erosion were higher in patients who received a new band at the time of the initial band removal (40%), compared to replacing it 3 or more months after the extraction (9%). In general, it is not recommended to place a new gastric band once erosion has occurred.

Esophageal complications

Esophagitis and reflux are infrequent complications following LAGB. Deflation of the band and acid-suppression therapy is the mainstay of treatment. However, if intractable to medical therapy, band removal or conversion to RYGB may be necessary.

Esophageal dilatation proximal to the band device has been observed in as many as 10% of patients. This so-called "pseudoachalasia syndrome" may develop when the band is excessively inflated or in the setting of excessive amounts of food intake. Pouch dilatation has also been associated with a history of binge eating behavior. Patients often present with food and saliva intolerance, reflux and epigastric discomfort. The diagnosis can be confirmed with an upper gastrointestinal (UGI) series. Initial treatment is removal of all fluid from the band along with behavioral diet modifications. This is usually successful in reversing esophageal dilatation, however, persistent dilatation will require band explant.

Hiatus hernia

Hiatus hernia is often a pre-existing but unrecognized condition in patients undergoing bariatric surgery. This can lead to ongoing intractable reflux necessitating reoperation or band removal. Thus, a simple crural repair can be performed at the initial operation to avoid these complications. A retrospective review of 1,298 patients who underwent LAGB alone and 520 patients who underwent LAGB with concurrent hiatal hernia repair showed that the rate of reoperation was significantly reduced in patients who had hiatal repair at the time of LAGB as compared with those who had LAGB alone (1.7 vs 5.6%, respectively).[11]

Port complications

Infection of the subcutaneous port occurs in about 1% of patients that undergo LAGB.[8] A trial of antibiotics can be attempted, but any signs of abscess or persistent infection will require the port to be removed with the connection tubing placed back into the peritoneal cavity. After 2–3 months, assuming that there are no signs of infection, a new port can be placed with tubing being retrieved laparoscopically. A late presentation of a port site infection should prompt investigation with EGD to rule-out possible band erosion.

Rotation of the port is much more common occurring in 3%–4% of patients, but this can be repositioned under local anesthesia. Other issues with the subcutaneous port such as disruption or leakage of the tubing are seen in 1%–2% of patients. Diagnosis is confirmed with contrast injected into the port under fluoroscopy visualization.

LSG

Hemorrhage

Bleeding after LSG can be attributed to a number of potential areas, with the staple line bleeding the most common; staple line bleeding can be either intra- or extra-luminal. Other potential areas include the gastroepiploic vessels, short gastric vessels, spleen and liver. Significant bleeding is a rare event ranging from 0.7%–3.3%.[12–13] The use of staple line reinforcement (SLR) to buttress the staple line is advocated by some to reduce the risk of bleeding. There have been several randomized controlled trials and comparative studies which report that SLR can decrease operative time by minimizing the need to clip or over-sew points of bleeding. Fortunately, postoperative bleeding is often self-limited, and can be treated with close monitoring, fluid resuscitation, discontinuation of any anti-coagulation medication, and transfusion of packed red blood cells as needed. Hemodynamically unstable patients who do not respond to transfusion should be taken back to the operating room for exploration. Drains placed in the area to monitor for postoperative bleeding can be ineffective and may be misleading.

Leak

Postoperative staple line leak is the one of the most dreaded complications after LSG. Leak rates are 1%–2% in most series,[12–14] but can be as high as 5%. Postoperative tachycardia, worsening abdominal pain, fever, tachypnea, hypoxia, hypotension and oliguria all can be signs of a leak, and diagnostic testing should be pursued to rule out a leak as soon as possible. UGI series is the study of choice for diagnosis, although a CT abdomen/pelvis may be useful as well. Leaks can be classified in several different ways; by the timing of presentation postoperatively, the degree of containment, or the location. Csendes *et al.*[15] classified leaks, although in RYGB data, as early (POD 1–3), intermediate (POD 4–7), or late (POD > 8). In terms of degree of containment based on radiologic study, a subclinical leak is one that is contained or controlled, and a clinical leak is disseminated with extrusion of contents into the abdominal cavity. Staple line leaks after LSG most commonly occur proximal at the angle of His near the gastroesophageal junction (EGJ),[13] but can occur anywhere along the staple line. Proximal leaks near the EGJ are more problematic as they tend to be more difficult to heal.

Prevention of leaks is an area with a large area of focus given the morbidity of the complication. Reinforcement of the staple line with either a buttressing material or over-sewing (serosa–serosa apposition — Lembert suture) the staple line is employed by most surgeons to decrease leaks. Bougie size is also associated with leak rates. A large meta-analysis of 9991 LSG cases reported that a smaller bougie (<40 French) was associated with a higher rate of staple-line leak (2.5% < 40 F, 1.7% 40–49 F, and 0.9% > 50 F).[16] The smaller bougie size is more likely to lead to narrowing near the angularis with resulting delayed emptying of the sleeve and higher intra-luminal gastric pressure contributing to staple-line leak.

Treatment of a staple-line leak after LSG is still an evolving field, but most of the focus has been centered on endoscopic stenting. Initial treatment of a leak is determined by the patients' hemodynamic stability and whether the leak is contained or not. Patients who are stable and have a contained leaked may be managed with a percutaneous drain. All other patients will require surgical intervention with peritoneal lavage, suture closure of staple line leak and wide drainage. Suture repair is often not possible or not effective given the high degree of inflammation associated with a staple line leak. Surgical exploration may be attempted laparoscopically but with a low threshold for conversion to open.[17] Once the leak is well-drained and controlled, endoscopic stenting can be attempted. Endoscopic stenting typically involves placing a fully-covered, self-expanding metal stent within the gastric sleeve to cover the area of leak, thereby diverting stomach contents away from the leak and allows for oral intake during the healing process. There is some uncertainty regarding the length of time that a stent should be left in prior to reimaging but 4–6 weeks is standard practice in most academic circles.[18] Initial reports are promising in regards to facilitating closure of the leak and decreasing hospital stay. Complications related to endoluminal stent placement include distal migration of the stent, epigastric pain, ulceration and bleeding. Endoscopic suturing devices have been used to secure the stent in an effort to minimize stent migration. In addition, improved longer stents are being developed which are specifically designed for the treatment of leaks after LSG.

Narrowing or stenosis

Clinically significant narrowing of the sleeve can be present at any time postoperatively, with patients presenting with PO intolerance, nausea, emesis, or dysphagia. Initially these symptoms may be related to early edema along the staple line, and will improve with time. However, if the symptoms do not improve, investigation with an UGI is needed to evaluate for technical issues related to the construction of the sleeve. Assessment should focus on emptying of the sleeve and any areas of narrowing. The most common technical reasons for the development of narrowing are aggressive over-sewing of the staple line and using a bougie that is too small. The area at greatest risk for narrowing is distal near the angularis incisura. The preferable bougie size is currently debated in the literature and can range from 30–60 French. In most cases, surgeons use a 36–40 French bougie for the sleeve construction and the larger sizes of bougies are reserved for when LSG is being performed as part of a staged procedure.

Management of stenosis should primarily consists of endoscopic dilation and or stenting, but surgical interventions such as seromyotomy, wedge resection, or conversion to a RYGB are also options.

A seromyotomy involves a longitudinal full-thickness incision across the stricture down to the gastric mucosa, a transverse repair and an optional omental patch to buttress the repair.[26] Another option to deal with the stricture is a wedge resection, which involves complete transection of the stomach at the level of the stricture, and a subsequent gastro-gastric anastomosis. However, there are no large series to date comparing these techniques and more studies are necessary to look into outcomes.

Laparoscopic RYGB

Leak

The leak rate after RYGB ranges from 2%–5%, with the gastrojejunostomy (GJ) being the most common site, followed by the jejunojejunostomy (JJ) and lastly the remnant stomach. It can be challenging to clinically diagnose a leak in bariatric patients owing to their body habitus, co-morbidities, as well as diagnostic testing limitations. High clinical suspicion of an intra-abdominal process should prompt immediate diagnostic testing, but operative management should never be delayed if signs of instability are present. Diagnostic testing includes UGI and or CT scan of the abdomen and pelvis. If possible, laparoscopic exploration is preferred as visualization is usually adequate, allows for complete surveillance of the operative field, and spares the patient the morbidity of a laparotomy incision. Identification of the leak, suture repair, abdominal washout, and wide closed suction drainage are the basic tenants of exploration. Consideration should also be giving to placing an enteric feeding tube either via a gastrostomy tube in the remnant stomach, or a jejunostomy tube in the common channel distal to the JJ. The stable patient can be safely managed conservatively with closed suction drainage, antibiotics, NPO, and total parenteral nutrition.

Bleeding

Similar to LSG, extra-luminal staple line bleeding is usually self-limited in nature and can be treated conservatively with supportive measures. Intra-luminal bleeding complications in the gastric pouch or near the gastro-jejunal anastomosis can be treated with endoscopic interventions, such as epinephrine and electrocautery. Bleeding from the remnant stomach can be more difficult to manage. Conventional endoscopy cannot reach given the length of many Roux limbs, however, double balloon push endoscopies have been successful in reaching the remnant and are able to treat bleeding.[19] Refractory bleeding or inability to access endoscopically may necessitate surgical intervention. Operatively, a gastrotomy can be made in the remnant stomach for visualization and endoscopically the biliopancreatic limb can be accessed. Last resort to control bleeding would involve remnant gastrectomy or a revision of the offending anastomosis.

GJ ulcer and strictures

Marginal ulcers are late complications that develop at the GJ, and although the pathophysiology behind marginal ulcers is unclear, this is a common complication with an incidence of 4.6%.[20] Patients present with epigastric pain, food intolerance, nausea, or emesis, and can have varying degrees of chronicity. Endoscopy is diagnostic, showing ulcerative disease at the anastomosis or the mucosa of the jejunum. Patients typically respond well to proton pump inhibitor therapy, but a small percentage may require operative revision of the GJ anastomosis. Perforation of a marginal ulcer is very rare (<1%), but is a surgical emergency and will require resection and revision of the anastomosis.

Narrowing at the GJ can occur immediately after surgery, if not related to postoperative edema, it is usually secondary to a technical complication. An UGI exam can demonstrate severe narrowing of even failure of contrast to past into the jejunum. Depending on the level of narrowing this may require immediate surgical correction of the GJ. Patients with late strictures can present with nausea, non-bilious emesis, pain or food intolerance. Workup usually starts with an UGI, and subsequent EGD. A GJ stricture is defined as the inability to pass a 9-mm endoscope through the GJ anastomosis without resistance. GJ strictures respond well to through-the-scope (TTS) balloon dilation. Repeat TTS balloon dilation may be required in some cases. Strictures that are not responsive to TTS balloon dilation will require surgical revision.

Internal hernias

Internal hernias can present either early or late and almost always require emergent surgical intervention. Early hernias are almost always a technical complication related to the initial operation. Late hernias are more common, usually occurring around 1 year postoperatively, when the patient has had a significant amount of weight loss. The hernia can occur either through the mesojejunal defect, the space between the Roux and the BP limb (Peterson's defect), or through the transverse mesocolon defect in a retro-colic Roux limb. Patients present with signs and symptoms consistent with intestinal obstruction; nausea, emesis, abdominal pain, distension, obstipation and constipation. Patients may present in extremis; simultaneous resuscitation, NGT decompression, and preparation for operative intervention are necessary. Diagnosis is made clinically, but CT abdomen and pelvis with oral and IV contrast is usually confirmatory. CT findings may include a swirled appearance of mesenteric fat or vessels, tubular distal mesenteric fat surrounded by bowel loops, small-bowel obstruction, clustered loops of small bowel, small bowel other than duodenum posterior to the superior mesenteric artery, and right-sided location of the JJ anastomosis.

Operative management involves at least reduction of the internal hernia and closure of the potential space, but may require resection of any compromised bowel and possible re-anastomosis. Reduction of the herniated small intestine is best accomplished by identifying the ileocecal valve and reducing the bowel in a hand-over-hand matter from distal to proximal. Based on the patient's operative findings it may be necessary to establish enteric access via a feeding jejunostomy tube.

Intussusception

Although a rare complication, intussusception should be considered on the differential as a potential cause for intestinal obstruction after RYGB. The most often affected site involves the common
channel with the JJ acting as a lead point. Intussusception can be
confidently diagnosed on CT because of its virtually pathognomonic
appearance. It appears as a complex soft tissue mass, consisting of
the outer intussuscipiens and the central intussusceptum. There is
often an eccentric area of fat density within the mass representing
the intussuscepted mesenteric fat, and the mesenteric vessels are
often visible within it. A rim of orally administered contrast medium
is sometimes seen encircling the intussusceptum, representing
coating of the opposing walls of the intussusceptum and the intussuscipiens. The intussusception will appear as a sausage-shaped mass
when the CT beam is parallel to its longitudinal axis, but will appear
as a "target" mass when the beam is perpendicular to the longitudinal axis of the intussusceptions.

Due to the rare occurrence of jejunal intussusception, there are
no large prospective studies for surgical treatment. Reduction of the
affected limb will treat the acute obstruction, but resection of
the affected segment has been recommended as it appears to lead
to fewer recurrences.[22]

Gastro-gastric (GG) fistula

In the earlier RYGB experience, GG fistulas were very common in
partially divided or undivided remnants, however, as completely
divided (isolated) RYGBs are now standard, GG fistulas are much
rarer. A large series reported the incidence of GG fistula after RYGB
to be 1.2%.[23] An upper GI with water-soluble contrast showing flow
of contrast into the remnant stomach is the study of choice, but
EGD can also be diagnostic. Patients often present with weight
regain and are asymptomatic. Some patients may present with pain
from a GJ ulcer secondary to increased acid exposure from the gastric remnant. Asymptomatic patients with good retention of weight
loss do not necessarily require surgical intervention. Laparoscopic

revision with remnant partial gastrectomy (including the GG fistula) has been shown to be effective and safe.[24]

Conclusion

Complications and mortality following surgical treatment of severe obesity vary based upon the procedure performed. Overall 30-day mortality for bariatric surgical procedures is <1 percent. Mortality rates are higher in men than in women and for those aged 65 and older. Both in-hospital and 30-day mortality are decreased when bariatric surgery is performed by surgeons and hospitals that perform more than 100 procedures a year. The most common causes of early re-hospitalization are nausea, vomiting, and dehydration, abdominal pain and wound problems. The most common causes of early mortality are pulmonary emboli and complications related to leaks. RYGB complications are diverse and include gastrointestinal leak, bleeding, GJ ulcer, GJ stricture, cholelithiasis, ventral hernias and internal hernias. Some complications are seen during the early postoperative periods while others may present weeks to months following the surgery. LAGB Bariatric Complicationscomplications include band erosion, band slippage, port malfunction, esophageal dilatation and esophagitis, LSG complications include staple line leaks, bleeding, narrowing or stenosis of the sleeve and reflux.

References

1. Birkmeyer NO, Dimick JB, Share D *et al.* (2010) Hospital complication rates with bariatric surgery in michigan. *JAMA* **304**(4): 435-442.
2. Murr M *et al.* (2007) A state-wide review of contemporary outcomes of gastric bypass in Florida. *Ann Surg* **245**: 699–706.
3. Saunders J *et al.* (2008) One-year readmission rates at a high volume bariatric surgery center: Laparoscopic adjustable gastric banding, laparoscopic gastric bypass, and vertical banded gastroplasty-Roux-en-Y gastric bypass. *Obes Surg* **18**(10): 1233–1240.
4. Brethauer SA (2013). ASMBS updated position statement on prophylactic measures to reduce the risk of venous thromboembolism in bariatric surgery patients. *Surg Obes Relat Dis.* **9**(4): 493–497.

5. Casella G *et al.* (2010) A time-saving technique for specimen extraction in sleeve gastrectomy. *World J Surg* **34**: 765–767.
6. Warschkow R *et al.* (2013) Concomitant cholecystectomy during laparoscopic Rouxen-Y gastric bypass in obese patients is not justified: a meta-analysis. *Obes Surg.* **23**(3): 397–407.
7. Lee DY *et al.* (2013) The incidence of trocar-site hernia in minimally invasive bariatric surgery: A comparison of multi vs single-port laparoscopy. *Surg Endosc* **27**: 1287–1291.
8. Chevalier JM *et al.* (2004) Complications after laparoscopic adjustable gastric banding for morbid obesity: Experience with 1,000 patients over 7 years. *Obes Surg* **14**(3): 407–414.
9. Pieroni S *et al.* (2010) The "O" Sign, a simple and helpful tool in the diagnosis of laparoscopic adjustable gastric band slippage. *Am J Roentgenol* **195**: 1, 137–141.
10. Brown, WA *et al.* (2013) Erosions after laparoscopic adjustable gastric banding. *Ann Surg* **257**(6): 1047–1052.
11. Gulkarov I *et al.* (2008) Hiatal hernia repair at the initial laparoscopic adjustable gastric band operation reduces the need for reoperation. *Surg Endosc* **22**(4): 1035–1041.
12. Lalor, P *et al.* (2008) Complications after laparoscopic sleeve gastrectomy. *Surg Obes Relat Relat Dis* **4**: 33–38.
13. Mittermair R. (2013) Results and complications after laparoscopic sleeve gastrectomy. *Surgery today.* September, Epub.
14. Seiber P *et al.* (2013) Five-year results of laparoscopic sleeve gastrectomy. *Surg Obes Relat Dis* July, Epub.
15. Csendes A *et al.* (2005) Conservative management of anastomotic leaks after 557 open gastric bypasses. *Obes Surg* **15**: 1252–1256.
16. Parikh M *et al.* (2013) Surgical strategies that may decrease leak after laparoscopic sleeve gastrectomy. *Ann Surg* **257**: 231–237.
17. Rebibo L *et al.* (2012) Early gastric fistula after laparoscopic sleeve Gastrectomy: Surgical management. *J Visceral Surg* **149**: 319–324.
18. Bhayani N, Swanstrom, L. (2013) Endoscopic therapies for leaks and fistulas after bariatric surgery. *Surg Innov*, Epub.
19. Dick A *et al.* (2010) Gastrointestinal bleeding after gastric bypass surgery: Nuisance or catastrophe? *Surg Obes Relat Dis* **6**: 643–647.
20. Coblijn UK *et al.* (2013) Development of ulcer disease after Roux-en-Y Gastric Bypass, incidence, risk factors, and patient presentation: A systematic review. *Obes Surg*, Epub.

21. Hamdan K *et al.* (2011) Management of late postoperative complications of bariatric surgery. *Brit J Surg* **98**: 1345–1355.
22. Daellenbach L *et al.* (2011) Jejunojejunal intussusception after Roux-en-Y gastric bypass: A review. *Obes Surg* **21**(2): 253–263.
23. Carrodeguas L *et al.* (2005) Management of gastrogastric fistulas after divided Roux-en-Y gastric bypass surgery for morbid obesity: Analysis of 1292 consecutive patients and review of literature. *Surg Obes Relat Dis*; **1**(5): 467–474.
24. Salimath J *et al.* (2009) Laparoscopic remnant Gastrectomy as a novel approach for treatment of gastrogastric fistula. *Surg Endosc* **23**: 2591–2595.
25. Finks JF *et al.* (2012) Predicting risk for venous thromboembolism with bariatric surgery: results from the Michigan Bariatric Surgery Collaborative. *Ann Surg*; **255**(6): 1100–1104.
26. Vilallonga R *et al.* (2013). Laparoscopic Management of Persistent Strictures After Laparoscopic Sleeve Gastrectomy. *Obes Surg.* **23**: 1655–1661.

Chapter 8

Innovations in Bariatric Surgery

George Pontikis,* Pornthep Prathanvanich[†] and Bipan Chand[†,‡]

*Department of Surgery, Loyola University
Medical Center, Maywood, Illinois
†Department of Surgery, Stritch School of Medicine
Loyola University, Chicago

In balancing the risks of surgery and the associated co-morbidities of obesity with the risk reduction associated with weight loss, the National Institute of Health has recommended bariatric surgery in the following individuals: Those diagnosed with Class III obesity (BMI > 40 kg/m²), or Class II obesity (BMI = 35–39.9 kg/m²) with co-morbid conditions, when dietary and lifestyle modifications have failed. Certainly, the most common bariatric procedures performed are laparoscopic Roux-en-Y gastric bypass (LRYGB), adjustable gastric band (LAGB) and sleeve gastrectomy (LSG). Several recent studies have demonstrated stable long-term outcomes, with 61–68% excess weight loss (EWL) in LRYGB, 47–50% EWL in LAGB and 56–60% in LSG.[1,2] Despite the promising results regarding weight loss, these procedures can result in several well-known complications, particularly in patients with BMI > 60 or morbid obesity with severe co-morbidities. Malabsorptive surgeries possess the risk for dumping syndrome, anastomotic disruption or leak in 0%–7%, anastomotic

---

‡Corresponding author.

stricture and long-term nutritional deficiencies in 3–22%, while LAGB is associated with band slippage, erosion and ulcer. Taking these risks and complications into account, this should encourage further and continued development of less invasive techniques and devices as either primary, adjunct, or bridging therapies, mimicking the effects of conventional bariatric surgery on weight and co-morbidities with the hope of minimizing these undesired side effects.[6] The American Society for Gastrointestinal Endoscopy (ASGE) and The American Society for Metabolic and Bariatric Surgery (ASMBS) recommend that for any non-primary weight loss procedures (e.g. bridging or metabolic surgery) a minimum threshold of 5% total body weight lost should be attained, as this has demonstrated significant reduction in diabetes and cardiovascular risk factors dyslipidemia in association with morbid obesity.

To facilitate the development of minimally invasive techniques that mimic the effects of bariatric surgery, one must understand the anatomic adjustments made to facilitate weight loss: (1) Gastric restriction through isolation of the gastric cardia, (2) exclusion of the distal stomach from alimentary flow, (3) exclusion of the proximal small bowel from alimentary flow, (4) exposure of the jejunum to partially digested nutrients, (5) delivery of partially digested nutrients to the distal intestine and (6) partial vagotomy. The aim of this chapter is to provide an overview of the latest minimally invasive techniques, mimicking conventional bariatric surgery. Both surgical procedures and less invasive endoscopic bariatric therapies (EBT) can be categorized according to their intended mechanism of action:

1. Restrictive procedure
   1.1 Space occupying devices: Intragastric balloons (IGBs) (e.g. BIB, Heliosphere BAG, Spatz Adjustable Balloon System (ABS))
   1.2 Gastric restrictive methods (Gastric plication/partition: TOGA, BaroSense, SurgASSIST, Endocinch, TERIS)
2. Malabsorptive methods:
   2.1 Endoscopic duodenal–jejunal sleeve (Endobarrier)
   2.2 Gastroduodenal–jejunal sleeve (Valentx)

3. Techniques potentially influencing gastric function
   3.1 Gastric botulinum toxin
   3.2 Gastric pacing
   3.3 Vagal nerve stimulation (VNS)

Most of the procedures are EBT except gastric pacing and VNS, which require laparoscopy.

IGBs

The use of endoscopic IGBs in surgical weight loss originated from its initial use in psychiatric patients with gastric bezoars in 1982. The first set of balloons were constructed from gum and latex and have since evolved to smooth, spherical, saline-filled or air-filled silicone devices (e.g. BioEnterics intragastric balloon, BIB, Allergan, Irvine, CA, USA; Heliosphere balloon, Heliosphere BAG, Heliscopie, Vienne, France), with some even allowing for volume adjustments (Spatz ABS, Jericho, NY, USA). The objective in IGB placement is to restrict gastric volume and induce early satiety with a temporary device placed endoscopically under conscious sedation. The IGB should be removed after a maximum of six months, due to the risk of spontaneous balloon deflation and increased risk of esophagitis, gastroesophageal reflux, gastric mucosal erosion, ulcer and small bowel obstruction. The primary indications are morbid obesity with severe co-morbidities or super morbid obesity, with IGB insertion serving as a bridging therapy to reduce anesthesia and surgical risks prior to definitive bariatric surgery. Success with IGB therapy predicts success with subsequent restrictive bariatric procedures. In contrast, malabsorptive procedures are offered to patients in whom IGB therapy did not result in appreciable pre-operative weight loss. Absolute contraindications to the placement of IGBs include previous gastric surgery, hiatal hernia of 5 cm or greater and the presence of known lesions of the upper gastrointestinal tract.

Machytka E *et al.*[3] reported 18 patients with mean BMI of 37.3 were implanted with the Spatz ABS for 12 months with an average of 24.4 kg or 48.8% EWL at 52 weeks. Implantation times varied from

8–60 m. They also demonstrated that with the Spatz adjustable balloon, patients safely continued to lose weight beyond 6 months. However, 5 of 18 balloons (28%) were removed after short duration (6–28 weeks) secondary to device related issues, including inflation tube or balloon leaks, valve defects, erosive gastritis and Mallory–Weiss tears.

From another retrospective analysis of 2,515 patients with a mean BMI of 44.8 ± 7.8 kg/m^2 who underwent endoscopic placement of IGB, only 2 (0.08%) were unsuccessful/.[4] At 6-month follow-up, the %EWL was 33.9±18.7. The patients demonstrated significant improvements in diabetes and hypertension in 86.9% and 93.7%, respectively. The authors reported a complication rate of 2.8%.

The main concern of IGBs is weight recidivism after removal. Several studies found that 28%–80% of patients demonstrated complete recidivism of their procedure-related weight loss after one year. Two years after removal, >10% EWL is maintained by 24–47% of patients.[4] Forlano R *et al.*[5] demonstrated the long-term results of patients after removal of IGBs. They studied 130 obese patients with a mean BMI of 43 kg/m^2 who underwent IGB insertion and was maintained for a six month period. The mean weight and BMI decreased by 13.2 kg and 5.1 kg/m^2 respectively. The mean glycemia, insulinemia, Homeostasis Model Assessment index, triglyceridemia and alanine aminotransferase levels were significantly reduced at six months after IGB insertion. After a median follow-up of 22 months from IGB removal, 50% of responders maintained or continued to lose weight. They concluded that placement of an IGB resulted in a positive effect on weight reduction and an associated improvement in insulin sensitivity, hepatic steatosis and features of the metabolic syndrome in 76% of patients. In the US, IGBs have not yet been approved for wide use and are still waiting randomized controlled trials and long-term data to demonstrate its effectiveness as a proven weight loss procedure.

Gastric Restrictive Methods

Given the limited durability of a temporary prosthesis, the development of endoscopic suturing and stapling soon occurred. At present time, there are numerous devices in various stages of development to perform vertical gastric plication, transoral/endoscopic plication or partition procedures aimed in creating a restrictive gastric pouch/conduit. The current generation of endoscopic gastric volume restriction devices requires significant skill and time compared to implantable space-occupying procedures. With continuing device development and improvement, the goal is to increase user-friendliness while decreasing the steep learning curve associated with these innovative technologies.

1. *Endoscopic stapling*

Transoral gastroplasty (TOGA) (TOGA System; Satiety, Inc, Palo Alto, Calif) is the first endoscopic stapling device to create full-thickness apposition. Using a strictly endoluminal approach, TOGA creates a stapled gastric sleeve pouch along the lesser curvature of the stomach. Two pilot studies assessing the TOGA system in the treatment of obesity in humans have been published. The initial feasibility of this technique in 33 human subjects was reported by Moreno *et al.* and Deviere *et al.*[2,4] In both studies, this treatment method was effective with respect to weight loss, quality of life improvement and safety. The mean EWL was 24.4%–46% at 6 months. The most commonly reported adverse effects were transient epigastric pain, nausea, vomiting, dysphagia, throat pain and esophagitis; however, most of these symptoms resolved spontaneously or with pharmacological treatment. At six months, endoscopy demonstrated a fully or partially persistent gastroplasty in all patients. Deviere *et al.*[2] also reported improvement in hemoglobin A1C levels, lipid levels and an overall reduction in hypertension. Although this method appears to be an effective and safe treatment for obesity, additional multicenter and randomized studies are necessary before its widespread implementation. The larger phase III study did not meet the FDA requirements and eventually the device and company became dismantled.

2. *Endoluminal vertical gastroplasty (EVG) or Transoral gastric volume reduction (TGVR)*

In 2008, Fogel *et al.*[2,4] first described the use of the Bard Endo-Cinch Suturing System (C. R. Bard, Inc, Murray Hill, NJ) under general anesthesia for the treatment of obesity in 64 patients. Seven sutures were deployed in a continuous and cross-linked fashion from the proximal fundus to the distal body. Once the suture is fixed, distention of the stomach is significantly limited. Patients had a significant reduction in BMI at 12 months (mean [SD] BMI 39.9 ± 5.1 kg/m^2 vs 30.6 ± 4.7 kg/m^2; $p < 0.001$) and a percentage of excess weight loss (%EWL) of 21.1, 39.6 and 58.1 at 1, 3 and 12 months, respectively. Only 14 patients underwent repeat endoscopy between 3 and 12 months post-procedure to assess the suture line. Of the 14 patients, 11 remained completely or partially intact and did not require additional intervention. There were minimal complications reported such as vomiting and reflux-like symptoms after procedure, most of which self-resolved within 24 h. No patients were reported to have any serious adverse events and no overnight observations were required. In 2012, Brethauer SA *et al.* presented an early prospective trial of an endoscopic suturing gastroplasty technique for the treatment of morbid obesity.[7] Eighteen patients underwent the procedure at 2 institutions. Using an updated version of the EndoCinch (Bard Medical, Murray Hill, NJ): The RESTORe (Randomized Evaluation of Endoscopic Suturing Transorally for Anastomotic Outlet Reduction) Suturing System (RSS) device (Bard/Davol, Warwick, RI) to approximate the anterior and posterior walls of the stomach, an average of six sutures were placed. While the device used by Fogel *et al.* implemented a continuous suture pattern, the RSS device employed an interrupted pattern to create the plication. All patients underwent general anesthesia with an average operative time of 2 h. The RSS study found that only 50% of their patients (7/14) demonstrated significant weight loss (>30% EWL) at 12 months; however, patients had a significant reduction in BMI at 12 months (mean [SD] BMI 38.6 ± 4.2 kg/m^2 vs 36.0 ± 4.8 kg/m^2; $p = 0.006$) and EWL of 22.8%, 29.9% and 27.7% at 1, 3 and 12 months, respectively. At 1 month post-procedure, only 2 patients had all sutures intact and by 12 months nearly all the sutures had pulled free. Well-designed studies with sham controlled trials and long-term follow-up will be needed to measure the durability of the observed weight loss. The stability of the gastric sutures remains unproven given the lack of long-term data. Certainly, technological improvements and increasing experience will enhance outcomes and the ability to perform this procedure competently.

Malabsorptive Methods

The main principle behind conventional bariatric surgery involves exclusion of the duodenum and proximal jejunum and exposure of the distal jejunum to undigested nutrients. The two new endoluminal bypass procedures were developed in animal models, simulating proximal small intestinal bypass without actual changes in anatomy.

1. *Endoscopic duodenojejunal bypass sleeve*

DJBS Endobarrier (GI dynamics Inc., Lexington, MA, USA) is an endoscopic method used to reduce jejunal absorption. This was the first device of its kind with a 60 cm single use impermeable fluoropolymer sleeve that is anchored in the duodenal bulb with a self-expanding nickel-titanium alloy (Nitinol) anchor extending into the proximal jejunum. Therefore gastric content passes through the interior while pancreatic and biliary juices pass alongside the exterior of the sleeve. These procedures generally take place under general anesthesia and are completed in 15–45 m; however, these procedures can also be performed under conscious sedation. In the first reported human series, the DJBS was successfully deployed in 12 patients with a mean 23.6% EWL after 12 weeks. A second human series was reported with 25 patients and found an EWL of 22% after 12 weeks, a mean EWL of 22% compared to 5% EWL in a diet modification control group. Most complications, such as abdominal pain, nausea and vomiting, were transient and encountered during the first week after implantation.[2,4] Several more serious adverse events were also encountered over a longer period of time, including hematemesis, sleeve migration, obstruction and mucosal tears (an oropharyngeal and an esophageal mucosal tear). Fortunately, all complications were managed conservatively, endoscopically, or by retrieval of the device. The device demonstrated inhibitory effects on satiety as well as improvements in co-morbid conditions such as DM, hypertension and hyperlipidemia. Appreciable reductions in fasting blood glucose, insulin and HbA1c (–2.1%) were observed. Although this device has been primarily used as a bridge therapy to surgery for the super morbidly obese population, preliminary studies are showing convincing evidence to use this as a therapeutic modality for resistant obesity-induced diabetic patients. Long-term follow-up data for while the device is in place and after removal is not yet available. Future studies are needed to clarify the safety and durability of the DJBS.

2. *Endoscopic gastroduodenal-jejunal sleeve*

The ValenTx (ValenTx Inc, Carpinteria, CA, USA), is another implantable and removable sleeve launched in 2011 and placed by a combination of endoscopy and laparoscopy. This device is twice as long as the Endobarrier (120 cm vs 60 cm) and also bypasses the stomach. While a self-expanding anchor in the duodenum characterizes the Endobarrier, the ValenTx device is laparoscopically attached to the distal esophagus. During the procedure, the gastroesophageal junction is dissected at the level of the diaphragmatic hiatus and eight full-thickness suture anchors secure the polyester cuff. The only published three-month trial demonstrated that 17 out of 22 implanted patients (77%) maintained the device, reaching an average of 40% EWL. Improvement in glycemic status was achieved in all seven diabetic patients. After three months, the 17 sleeves that remained *in situ* varied with respect to their length left in the stomach. Of the total 120 cm length of the device, 10–40 cms was found to reside in the stomach with the remainder of the device lying in the duodenum and proximal jejunum. This device is usually removed after 3 months of treatment. Short and long-term follow-up data as well as data after removal are yet to be investigated.

Gastric Botulin Toxin Injection

Botulinum toxin blocks the release of acetylcholine from the neuron and is used in the management of muscular and glandular overactivity. In humans, endoscopic injections with botulinum toxin has led to conflicting results, potentially due to differences in the location of administration (antrum and/or fundus region), variance in doses of the toxin and patient selection. Most studies show no effect of botulinum toxin injections in the antrum alone. In contrast, injections in both fundus and antrum seem to be more effective. One of the most positive randomized, double blind studies, Li L *et al.*[2] showed twice as much weight loss in botulinum toxin treated patients than in saline injected controls after 2 months; however, none of the studies have follow up any longer than four months and overall results do not appear convincing. The potential effects of botulinum injections in weight loss therefore remain disputable and are not currently offered as a permanent solution for obesity.

Gastric Pacing

Laparoscopic implantable gastric stimulation devices generate electrical pulses via bipolar leads along the lesser curvature. Performed while under general anesthesia, these leads are placed into the seromuscular layer of the gastric wall and are connected to a generator that is positioned subcutaneously along the abdominal wall. The first set of results in obese patients demonstrated that gastric pacing induces a reduction in appetite and enhanced level of satiety. Non-randomized trials with a follow-up time between 10–24 months reported 20–40% EWL in a total of 500 severely obese patients (BMI > 40 kg/m^2). The most important but less encouraging results derived from two prospective, randomized, placebo-controlled, double blind trials: The O-01 trial and Screened Health Assessment and Pacer Evaluation (SHAPE) trial. In both studies, 12% EWL was reported in both treatment and control groups after 1 year. Some patients lost significant weight, while others showed little to no response to therapy. The complications usually described in association with this procedure include partial or complete dislodgment of the leads and more rarely, perforations of the stomach during lead implantation. Gastric pacing remains an interesting technique; however, optimal stimulation patterns, underlying mechanism and the effect on co-morbid conditions are yet to be elucidated. Currently, there is insufficient scientific evidence to support gastric pacing as a suitable treatment for obesity.

VNS

VNS is delivered by an electrode placed subcutaneously that provides electric stimulation to the vagus nerve (e.g. EnteroMedics VBLOC, St. Paul, MN, USA). This technique was first indicated in epilepsy and therapy-resistant depression. In recent studies involving pigs, rats and obese mini-pigs, vagal pacing diminished overall food intake and provided a reduction in weight and fat mass, indicating a role in satiety signaling. VNS also increases energy expenditure by activating human brown adipose tissue (BAT). BAT activity is inversely correlated with BMI and body fat percentage as demonstrated by means of FDG-PET-CT (^{18}F-fluorodeoxyglucose positron-emission tomography and computed tomography). BAT show significantly higher energy expenditure as compared to subjects without BAT activity. This suggests BAT is related to the development of obesity and that increasing BAT activity could be a new treatment modality for obesity. Vijgen *et al.*[8] evaluated 15 patients undergoing VNS therapy (BMI = 25.2 ± 3.5 kg/m^2). Basal metabolic rate was significantly higher when VNS was turned on (mean change; +2.2%). Also, the change in energy expenditure upon VNS intervention strongly correlated to the change in BAT activity by FDG-PET-CT ($r = 0.935$, $p < 0.001$). An average reduction of 14–23% EWL after 6 months of VNS has been reported ($n = 53$). Other studies found an average weight loss of 2 BMI points or 7 kg after one year. No serious adverse events have been encountered in the literature. Never the less, it is uncertain whether VNS can induce a definite sustainable therapeutic effect on obesity. Its potential clinical value as a target for therapy has yet to be confirmed in randomized controlled studies.

Metabolic Surgery

In 2013, The World Health Organization (WHO) found 347 million people were diagnosed with type 2 diabetes (DM) worldwide, including 23.6 million individuals of the US population. The American Diabetes Association estimates that nearly 21 million people in the U.S. have DM, with another 54 million considered to be pre-diabetics. The direct and indirect medical costs linked to diabetes have risen from $174 billion in 2007 to $245 billion in 2012, reflecting the medical and financial burden this disease places on our society. Along with the known medical therapies that exist to treat and control this disease, the curative effect of bariatric surgery on DM has forced the medical community to question the previous notion of the incurable nature of this disease.

In the US, over 170,000 bariatric surgeries are performed annually, with the literature demonstrating convincing evidence that these procedures are the superior method to provide patients both rapid and sustained weight loss. In concomitance with the appreciable reduction in BMI, recent studies have demonstrated the efficacy of bariatric surgery in alleviating other medical co-morbidities in association with morbid obesity. According to a landmark study published in the *Journal of the American Medical Association* (*JAMA*) in 2004, bariatric surgery has resulted in the remission of DM in 76.8%, elimination of hypertension in 61.7%, reduction in hypercholesterolemia in more than 70% and elimination of obstructive sleep apnea in 85.7% of patients. The focus in this section will be on the multifactorial mechanism that metabolic surgery provides in the treatment and resolution of DM. Several recent studies have evaluated the reduction in glucose levels by means of postoperative monitoring of the Hemoglobin A1c (HbA1c). These studies reported strikingly similar findings: 80%–90% of patients demonstrated normalization of the HbA1c to less than 7% by approximately 26 weeks after RYGB, with a mean HbA1c reduction of 3.8% at 2 years after surgery.

Many practitioners initially attributed the resolution of DM to decreased oral intake and expected weight loss. In contrast, the near immediate improvement of fasting glucose levels suggested a more intricate system of anatomic and physiologic derangements imposed by the surgery. This concept was initially validated in an animal model in which non-obese diabetic rats underwent duodenal–jejunal bypass (DJB). Independent of weight loss or caloric intake, the DJB group exhibited improved glucose homeostasis, suggesting a more elaborate foregut exclusion mechanism rather than a model solely focused on weight loss and decreased caloric intake. Upon restoration of normal anatomy in the DJB rats, they quickly returned to pre-operative impaired glucose tolerance levels. The results from this study brought forth the recognition of the "anti-incretin factors," which are a set of neurohormonal molecules that provide diabetogenic signals in the foregut and play a pivotal role in the resolution of DM after bariatric surgery.

Ghrelin is a gastrointestinal peptide hormone produced by the oxyntic glands of the fundus and cells lining the duodenum. Its function is primarily suppression of the insulin-sensitizing hormone adiponectin, blocking of hepatic insulin signaling and inhibition of insulin secretion. It is also involved in appetite and food consumption via direct modulation of the central nervous system hunger mechanism. In rodents, chronic ghrelin administration causes hyperphagia and increased adiposity and was similarly found to increase appetite and food intake in humans after the administration of peripheral ghrelin. After resection of the fundus in sleeve gastrectomy (SG) or creation of the gastric pouch in RYGB, there is an overall decrease in circulating ghrelin resulting in overall improvement of metabolic homeostasis.

Gastric–inhibitory peptide (GIP) is another important molecule produced by the K cells of the duodenum and is a potent stimulator of insulin secretion. After SG, the shorter and more direct path by which the bolus travels to reach the duodenum results in an increase in GIP, providing stimulation of insulin secretion providing the expected decrease in blood glucose levels. Other notable gastrointestinal neuroendocrine molecules include GLP-1 and Peptide YY, which are released by the L-cells of the gut and provide multiple anorectic actions that mediate weight loss effects. Recent studies have found that GLP-1 and PYY stimulate insulin synthesis and release in response to nutrient ingestion while inhibiting overall glucagon secretion. This theory was validated by the use of GLP-1 receptor antagonist, resulting in impaired glucose tolerance in the DJB rat group.

According to the American Society of Metabolic and Bariatric Surgeons, the current indications for bariatric surgery include BMI greater than 40 or BMI greater than 35 with at least two obesity-related co-morbidities including DM, hypertension, hyperlipidemia, obstructive sleep apnea, non-alcoholic fatty liver disease, osteoarthritis, or heart disease. Given the increasing understanding of the chemical changes that occur in association with bariatric surgery, the current focus in the literature is in expanding the indications for bariatric surgery beyond weight loss. Several preliminary studies have demonstrated the efficacy of gastric bypass in the treatment of non-severe obese (BMI less than 35) DM patients at longer follow-up after bariatric surgery, achieving comparable improvement and remission rates of DM as seen in well-established studies for morbidly obese patients. Significant advancements have been made over the last 20 years in understanding the physiologic changes that occur secondarily to the anatomic derangements of bariatric surgery. It is essential that research in this area continue to expand, in an effort to broaden the use of these well-tolerated and efficacious procedures, to treat and potentially cure patients of other debilitating and lifelong diseases.

Single Incision Laparoscopic Surgery (SILS)

Laparoscopy is an ever-evolving field with continued emphasis on developing the least invasive methods to perform the well-known open surgical procedures. SILS arose in the early 1990's with its initial uses in performing single incision cholecystectomy and appendectomy. The use of SILS in bariatric surgery is currently in its infancy, but it is rapidly gaining popularity and implementation.

LRYGB is the most popular method and gold standard, for weight loss surgery used in bariatric surgery, with an expected EWL of 60–70%. Traditional LRYGB is a complex surgery requiring multiple abdominal incisions for the placement of the multiple trocars used to perform the procedure. Although the traditional laparoscopic approach to RYGB is far more prevalent, there is an increase in the utilization of SILS. The primary benefit of SILS lies within its name: A single laparoscopic incision is used to perform the entire surgery. In comparing SILS to traditional laparoscopy, there is a significant decrease in the number of incisions resulting in possible decrease postoperative procedural pain, decreased risk of wound infection, decreased risk of incisional hernia and an overall better cosmetic result. This method is not without disadvantages, including a small and limited angle in which to work and potential for steep learning curve. Additionally, the hypertrophic left liver seen in patients with fatty liver disease often hinders the surgeon's view of the entire stomach, consequently making it very challenging to obtain adequate exposure. Despite these disadvantages, there is promise in using SILS as a more routine approach to RYGB in appropriate patients.

As these cases are being performed in increasing numbers, modifications to the procedures are already underway to increase the efficiency by which they are performed. The procedure begins with a 6 cm omega-shaped incision to allow more space between trocars and permits the surgeon to manipulate the instruments more easily. It is also important to understand that SILS cannot be safely and effectively used in all patients and needs precise patient selection in order to maximize the effectiveness of the procedure. SILS is not indicated in super-obese patients (BMI greater than 60), patients taller than 180 cm are also poor candidates as they possess abundant intra-abdominal fat pads and with their height, create a very long distance between the umbilicus and the gastric pouch, making the surgery very difficult to perform. It is currently recommended that this procedure be performed by experienced bariatric surgeons with over 400 LRYGB completed.

Preliminary studies have shown that SILS patients experienced significantly longer operative times, no difference in hospitalization or EWL. In a postoperative survey, patients who underwent SILS demonstrated a statistically significant elevation in the level of satisfaction with the surgery and overall cosmetic result as compared to the patients undergoing the traditional procedure. SILS appears to be a feasible alternative to traditional laparoscopic bariatric procedures in select patients as demonstrated in early studies. With improvement in instrumentation and technological advances, the use of SILS will gain increasing popularity and will likely be widely implemented in the field of minimally invasive surgery.

References

1. ASGE/ASMBS (2011) Task Force On Endoscopic Bariatric Therapy. *Gastrointest Endosc* **74**(5): 943–953.
2. Siergiejko AS, Wróblewski E, Dabrowski A. (2011) Endoscopic treatment of obesity. *Can J Gastroenterol* **25**(11): 627–633.
3. Machytka E, Klvana P, Kornbluth A *et al.* (2011) Adjustable intragastric balloons: A 12-month pilot trial in endoscopic weight loss management. *Obes Surg* **21**: 1499–1507.
4. Verdam FJ, Schouten R, Greve JW *et al.* (2012) An update on less invasive and endoscopic techniques mimicking the effect of bariatric surgery. *J Obes* 1–10.
5. Forlano R, Ippolito AM, Iacobellis A *et al.* (2010) Effect of the bioenterics intragastric balloon on weight, insulin resistance, and liver steatosis in obese patients. *Gastrointest Endosc* **71**: 927–933.
6. Thompson CC, Chand B, Chen YK *et al.* Endoscopic suturing for transoral outlet reduction increases weight loss after roux-en-y gastric bypass surgery. *Gastroenterol* **145**: 129–137.
7. Brethauer SA, Chand B, Schauer PR *et al.* (2012) Transoral gastric volume reduction as intervention for weight management: 12-month follow-up of trim trial. *Soard* **8**(3): 296–303.
8. Vijgen GHE, Bouvy ND, Leenen L *et al.* (2013) Vagus nerve stimulation increases energy expenditure: Relation to brown adipose tissue activity. *Plos One* **8**(10): 1–8.
9. de la Cruz-Muñoz N, Messiah SE, Arheart KL *et al.* (2011) Bariatric surgery significantly decreases the prevalence of type 2 diabetes mellitus and pre-diabetes among morbidly obese multiethnic adults: Long-term results. *J Am Coll Surg*, **212**: 505–511.
10. Pirolla Eduardo H, Ricardo J, Mario L *et al.* (2012) A modified laparoscopic sleeve gastrectomy for the treatment of diabetes mellitus type 2 and metabolic syndrome in obesity. *Am J Surg* **203**(6): 785–792.
11. Lee WJ, Chong K, Chen CY *et al.* (2011) Diabetes remission and insulin secretion after gastric bypass in patients with body mass index <35 kg/m^2. *Obes Surg* **21**: 889–895.

12. Parikh M, Reda I, Dorice V *et al.* (2013) Role of bariatric surgery as treatment for type 2 diabetes in patients who do not meet current NIH criteria: A systematic review and meta-analysis. *J Am Coll Surg* **217**(3): 527–532.
13. Karra E, Ahmed Y, Batterham RL. (2010) Mechanisms facilitating weight loss and resolution of type 2 diabetes following bariatric surgery. *Trends Endocrin Met* **21**(6): 337–344.
14. Lanzarini E, Csendes A, Lembach H *et al.* (2010) Evolution of type 2 diabetes mellitus in non-morbid obese gastrectomized patients with Roux en-Y reconstruction: Retrospective study. *World J Surg* **34**: 2098–2102.
15. Huang CK, Yao SF, Lo CH *et al.* (2010) A novel surgical technique: Single-incision transumbilical laparoscopic Roux-en-Y gastric bypass. *Obes Surg* **20**: 1429–1435.
16. Mittermair R. (2013) Transumbilical single-incision laparoscopic sleeve gastrectomy: Short-term results and technical considerations. *J Minim Access Surg* **9**(3): 104.

Chapter 9

Nutrition after Bariatric Surgery

Karen Buzby and Danielle Rosenfeld Staub

All candidates for bariatric surgery require preoperative nutrition education, in the form of medical weight management, to help them prepare for the immediate and long term diet and lifestyle changes needed after surgery. Following surgery, ongoing coordinated care, including monitoring of diet and nutrition status, is required to ensure health and weight goals are achieved and maintained. The principles of the postoperative diet progression, macro- and micronutrient requirements, prevention and management of diet related complications as well as strategies for successful weight loss are reviewed for the three most commonly performed bariatric procedures, the Roux-en-Y gastric bypass (RYGB), sleeve gastrectomy (SG) and adjustable gastric band (AGB).

Diet Goals

Nutrition after weight loss surgery (WLS) is focused on changing food selection and eating habits to produce successful weight loss and to prevent nutrition related complications. While differences may exist between bariatric programs regarding specific dietary recommendations and diet advancement, the goals of the postoperative diet can be clearly defined and are summarized in Table 1.[1,2,3]

Table 1:   Goals of the bariatric surgery diet.

- To regulate eating behaviors and select low caloric foods & beverages to promote weight loss and weight maintenance.
- To ensure adequate fluid intake to prevent dehydration.
- To consume high quality protein to maintain muscle mass, promote wound healing, maintain visceral protein stores and promote satiety.
- To maximize diet tolerance by slowly introducing solid food.
- To meet micronutrient needs with vitamin and mineral supplementation.
- To prevent food related postoperative complications.

Postoperative Nutrition Care and Diet Progression

Patients are typically NPO for 24 h after surgery with intravenous fluids providing adequate hydration. Some surgical protocols require a limited upper gastrointestinal contrast study evaluating staple line integrity to determine if a leak or obstruction is present before the patient starts a liquid diet.

Current clinical practice is to use a multistage diet progression beginning with liquids and gradually advancing to solid foods.[1,2,3,4] A sample five-stage bariatric surgery diet is outlined in Table 2.[3] The purpose of the texture progression is to allow for post-operative healing and to prevent gastrointestinal complications. More research is needed to determine if this slow advancement is more effective than introducing solid foods earlier with regards to the incidence of complications or the degree of weight loss.[5] The registered dietitian, in collaboration with the bariatric surgeon and multi-disciplinary team, should develop institution-specific protocols for diet advancement and patient education.[1]

The process of introducing liquid and food after WLS can be described as "relearning how to drink and eat." Some individuals find it challenging to meet even the minimum fluid and protein goals in the early postoperative period. As each stage of the bariatric diet is reviewed practical tips are presented to assist clinicians in providing dietary advice to patients.

Bariatric clear liquids

Oral fluids are usually started the day after surgery (Table 2: Stage I).[1,2] Patients should be instructed to take small sips of water or another clear liquid beginning with 1 ounce over a 15 min period. This slow pace of drinking helps patients adjust to the small size of the newly created gastric pouch (~30mL volume) or sleeve. More

Table 2: Bariatric diet: Stages I–V. (Adapted from Ref. 3)

Stage I: Bariatric clear liquid diet

Duration: 1–2 days.

Foods/Fluids: Non-carbonated, caffeine-free, sugar-free beverages including water, low fat broth, sugar-free popsicles, diet gelatin, decaf/herbal teas, artificially sweetened beverages and diluted 100% juice. Artificial sweeteners such as aspartame, saccharin, sucralose and stevia are acceptable.

Vitamin and Mineral Supplementation: None

Stage II: Bariatric high protein full liquid diet

Duration: 14 days; (Post-op week 1 & 2)

Foods/Fluids: Liquid low calorie modular protein supplements, low fat milk products and milk alternatives; strained milk-based soups or pureed pea or lentil soups, vegetable juice; some programs permit thin hot cereals, low fat/light yogurts on the full liquid diet while other program introduce these foods on the pureed diet.

Vitamin and Mineral Supplementation: Begin chewable or liquid supplements.

Stage III: Bariatric pureed diet

Duration: AGB and RYGB: 2 weeks; (Post-op week 3 & 4)

       SG: May require 3–4 weeks on the pureed diet (Post-op week 3–6)

Foods/Fluids: Blended or liquefied foods low in sugar and fat. Scrambled eggs and egg substitutes, pureed meat and beans; flaked, water packed tuna or salmon, and meat alternatives; yogurt, cottage cheese, soft cheeses, hot/cold cereal; pureed fruit or vegetables. Continue liquid low calorie protein supplements. Encourage the addition of protein powders or non-fat dry milk solids to fortify blended foods.

Vitamin and Mineral Supplementation: Continue chewable or liquid recommended supplements.

(Continued)

Table 2:   (*Continued*)

Stage IV: Bariatric soft diet

Duration: AGB: 14 days; (Post-op week 5 & 6)

RYGB: > 14 days (Post-op week 5 & 6, patients often remain on a soft diet for a longer period of time)

SG: Progress as tolerated

Foods/Fluids: Ground or chopped (pea-size pieces recommended) tender cuts of meat and poultry, fish, cooked beans/lentils, meat alternatives; low fat dairy products; well-cooked vegetables and canned fruit, soft fresh fruit without peels or skins; toasted whole grain bread and crackers as tolerated. Avoid gummy starches (pasta, refined bread products) and dry meats.

Vitamin and Mineral Supplementation: Continue chewable or liquid recommended supplements.

Stage V: Bariatric regular diet

Duration: Initiated approximately 2 months after surgery or when tolerated.

Foods/Fluids: Solid foods, healthy-whole foods; lean proteins; low fat dairy; fresh fruits and vegetables; whole grain bread and cereals.

Vitamin and Mineral Supplementation: Continue recommended supplements. Change to tablet or pill form (< 11 mm in width and length) as tolerated.

suggestions on beginning liquids are listed in Text Box 1: Practical tips for meeting fluid goals after WLS. In keeping with diet goals, beverages should be low-sugar or sugar-free to minimize the consumption of "empty" calories.[4]

The bariatric clear liquid diet does not supply adequate protein or vitamins and minerals. If clear liquids are required for more than 48 h a high protein, low residue nutritional supplement should be added along with appropriate multivitamin and mineral supplements as long as their use is not contraindicated.[2]

Bariatric high protein full liquids and the use of modular protein supplements

The high protein full liquid diet (Table 2: Stage II) has slightly more texture than clears and is started after the patient demonstrates tolerance to clear liquids for 2 meals or upon discharge from the

Text Box 1:	Practical tips for meeting fluid goals after WLS.
Important Points	**Instructions and Practical Tips**
Initial rate of drinking	• Use a 1 oz medicine cup to guide intake. • Consume 1 oz in 6 to 8 "sips". • Suggested rate is 1 oz over a period of 15 min.
Rate of fluid consumption	• Advance pace from 4 oz/hr to 6 oz/hr to 8 oz/hr • Continue to advance pace as tolerated until new "normal" is established.
Daily fluid goals	• 48–64 oz/day[1,3] increase as tolerated to 80–100 oz/day. • Clear liquids should account for half of fluid intake.
Beverage temperature	• Individual preferences & tolerance vary. • Try cold, room temperature and hot beverages.
Protein supplements	• Thickness of liquid influences pace of drinking. • If smell or sight is unappealing, use a covered cup. • Select a protein drink with a minimum of 15–20 g protein & < 200 kcal/8 oz serving.
Kitchen utensils & Equipment	• Use water bottles with graduated fluid ounces to pace consumption. • Get a beverage shaker for mixing protein supplements. • Measuring cups and spoons are needed for accurate food preparations and portion control. • Infant spoon and fork set helps to take small bites of food. • Blender or food processor needed to modify food texture. • Do not use a straw, use of a straw may over fill the pouch with liquid or air.

hospital. The calorie and protein content of a bariatric diet, including full liquids, is similar to a very low calorie diet (VLCD) which provides large amounts of protein and a limited amount of carbohydrate and fat. In the early post-operative period calorie intakes between 400 to 800 kcal/d have been observed.[5]

Modular protein supplements of high biological value are used to meet protein requirements. The "protein digestibility corrected amino acid score" (PDCAA score) is used to assess the overall quality of a protein by indicating the body's ability to use the product for protein synthesis.[2,6] Based on the PDCAA, supplements derived from complete proteins such as milk protein (casein or various whey fractions), egg white and soy protein should be recommended due to their high PDCAA score of 100%.[6] The use of collagen-based products should be limited and not used as the sole source of protein after WLS. Collagen does not contain adequate amounts of the nine indispensable amino acids (IAA) and is lacking tryptophan, even with the addition of casein or another complete protein, these products may not contain all of the IAA.[6] Practitioners should be aware that in the presence of IAA deficiency, loss of lean body mass can occur despite meeting daily protein goals.[2]

Whey protein is rapidly digested and contains high levels of branched-chain amino acids, especially leucine, which helps prevent lean tissue breakdown.[2,7] Whey protein concentrates contain lactose but whey protein isolates are lactose free. Products containing soy and other vegetable proteins are available for vegetarians or individuals not able to tolerate whey. The vitamin and mineral content of protein supplements vary considerably. Products that are considered meal replacements usually contain more micronutrients than simple protein products. To further illustrate product variability a selection of commercially available protein supplements are compared in Table 3. In general, protein drinks are designed to supplement a diet of mixed foods and their extended use as the primary source of dietary protein is not advised.

Patient compliance with the use of protein supplements may be influenced by product taste, smell and texture. Premixed protein supplements in ready-to-go containers offer convenience but usually cost more per serving. Using a protein powder is more economical but measuring and mixing is required before use. It is important for patients to find a palatable protein supplement within their budget before surgery.

Due to volume restrictions, the variable micronutrient content of protein drinks and the limited number of foods consumed, the postoperative diet does not provide all of the essential vitamins and minerals. Therefore, a multivitamin and mineral supplement should be started during the full liquid diet and continued lifelong. (Refer to

Table 3: Comparison of commercially prepared modular protein supplements per 8 fl oz (237 mL) or approximately 30 grams of protein powder.

Product and Manufacturer*	Protein (g/8 oz)	Carbohydrate (g/8 oz)	Calories (kcal/8 oz)	Protein Source	Micronutrients**
Liquid Products:					
Boost Glucose Control®/Nestlé Health Science	16	16	190	Milk protein concentrate, soy protein isolate, sodium caseinate, L-arginine	Contains 26 vitamins and minerals.
Ensure® High Protein/Abbott Nutrition	14	13	120	Milk protein concentrate, less than 2% calcium caseinate, soy protein isolate.	Contains 24 vitamins and minerals.
Muscle Milk®/Cyto Sport, Inc.	14	4.8	128	Calcium sodium caseinate, milk protein isolate.	Contains 20 vitamins and minerals.
Myoplex EAS® Original/Abbott Nutrition	20	9.4	141	Milk protein concentrate, pea protein concentrate	Contains 25 vitamins and minerals.
Isopure *Zero Carb*/Natures Best	16	0	64	Whey protein isolate.	None
New Whey Liquid Protein/New Whey Nutrition	88	4.2	369	Blend of collagen protein isolate, whey protein isolate, casein protein isolate.	None

(Continued)

Table 3: *(Continued)*

Product and Manufacturer*	Protein (g/8 oz)	Carbohydrate (g/8 oz)	Calories (kcal/ 8 oz)	Protein Source	Micronutrients**
Protein Powders: (~30g mixed with water)					
Designer Whey Protein Powder/ Designer Protein, LLC	18	6	100	rBGH-free whey protein concentrate, rBGH-free whey protein isolate.	Contains 4 B vitamins, plus calcium, magnesium and zinc.
Genisoy Soy Powder/ Downright Healthy Foods LP	14	18	130	Soy protein isolate.	Contains 19 vitamins and minerals.
Pea Protein Powder/ Now Foods	24	1	120	100% Pure, non–GMO pea protein isolate.	Contains iron
Rice Protein Powder/ NutriBiotic	24	2	120	Enzymatically processed rice protein from whole grain, sprouted brown rice.	Contains iron.
Hemp Protein Powder/Bob's Red Mill Natural Foods, Inc.	14	10	120	Hemp protein powder.	Contains iron.

* Nutrient information obtained from manufacturers website accessed on 15 September 2015. Vanilla flavor products evaluated when available.
** Multiple servings required to meet 100% RDA. Daily vitamin and mineral supplements are required to ensure micronutrients needs are met.

the section on micronutrient requirements for a detailed discussion of vitamin and mineral needs.)

Each diet stage with the exception of clear liquids as previously noted, is usually followed for two weeks, but the individual's ability to tolerate the current diet will determine if they are ready to advance to the next diet stage. The patient should record daily fluid and protein intake to make sure they are making progress toward dietary goals. While keeping a written log of protein and fluid is acceptable, the availability of free internet and smart phone based applications, such as MyFitnessPal.com, LoseIt.com or the Super-Tracker on MyPlate.gov make tracking all dietary nutrients very easy and efficient.

Bariatric purees

The pureed diet (Table 2: Stage III) gradually increases gastric residue while minimizing the likelihood of obstruction from a bolous of inadequately chewed foods. Pureed foods are blended or liquefied and range in texture and consistency.[2] While pureed foods from all food groups can be introduced, protein-containing foods should be consumed first.

Food volume is initially limited to ¼ cup or 2 oz per meal. More food may be tolerated however due to the reduced size of the gastric pouch or sleeve, patients are instructed to be very cautious and slowly increase meal size. Also liquids should be consumed between meals rather than with food.[1,4] Separating eating and drinking will help to maximize food intake during meals and prevent the possibility of rapid digestion of food from the pouch or sleeve. Overconsumption of food or liquid can cause nausea, vomiting or a feeling of tightness, pressure or pain in the chest. It is important that individuals learn to recognize their sign or signal of fullness and use these body signals to prevent overfilling of the gastric pouch. Other important changes to eating behaviors are listed in Text Box 2: Eating behavior guidelines for bariatric surgery.

Text Box 2:   Eating behavior guidelines for bariatric surgery.

Eating Behavior	Instructions & Practical Tips
Separate eating & drinking	• Stop drinking 30 minutes before meals & snacks. • Do not drink during meal or snack. • Resume drinking 30 to 45 minutes after eating.
Take small bites of food	• Cut food into pea–size pieces. • A bite of food should be no larger than the size of a dime.
Chew foods well	• Chew food 15 or more times until it is of semi-liquid consistency.
Pace of eating	• 20 to 30 minutes per meal. • Do not graze or go beyond 45 min for one meal.
Timing of meals	• Regulate eating habits to make time for 3 meals a day. • Add snacks as needed to increase protein intake.
Food selection	• Eat protein containing foods first (lean protein, low fat dairy & vegetable protein sources) before foods with only carbohydrates and fats.
Signs of fullness	• Always stop eating when sign or signal of fullness are recognized.
Food preparation	• Do not fry foods. • Use moist cooking methods. • Measure portion sizes. • Use a blender or food processor to prepare pureed foods.

Bariatric soft diet

The soft diet (Table 2: Stage IV) introduces food with more texture while minimizing the likelihood of food related complications. High biological value proteins including tender cuts of lean meat, poultry, fish, low fat or fat free dairy, soy products and other meat alternatives are emphasized. Since plant based proteins tend to be deficient in one or more IAA[8] individuals preferring a plant-based diet may require additional nutrition counseling to ensure his or her protein needs are met after surgery when a smaller volume of food is consumed.

As patients adapt to eating, liquid protein supplements may be phased out of the diet. The benefits of consuming protein-containing foods are increased satiety and better diet quality. However, if protein intake from food sources is suboptimal or if food intolerances contribute to inadequate protein intake, the continued use of modular nutritional supplements is warranted to continue to meet daily protein goals.

Bariatric regular diet

Regular texture foods are appropriate for bariatric patients who are 2 or more months post-surgery[2,3] (Table 2: Stage V). In order to control calorie intake and promote optimal weight loss, protein-rich nutrient dense foods continue to be emphasized.

With the focus on protein, fruit and vegetable consumption may be limited in the first year after WLS. Over time, as calorie intake increases, fruits and vegetables are a good dietary option for proper weight maintenance. Recommendations for complex carbohydrates including cereals and grains should be individualized, since doughy or sticky carbohydrates may be poorly tolerated. (Refer to the section on diet-related gastrointestinal complications for a discussion of food intolerances.) Healthy dietary fats with n-3 fatty acids, such as olive oil and canola oil should be emphasized in moderation due to the calorie density of fat.

Table 4 outlines a sample 1200-calorie maintenance diet.[9] Continuing nutrition education should focus on the importance of avoiding high-calorie foods, such as fats (butter, cream, fried foods), sweets and beverages containing sugar. Patients who successfully avoid these foods consistently demonstrate satisfactory maintenance of weight loss after surgery.[10]

It is recommended to establish regular meal times and divide food up into 3 meals and snacks, as needed, in order to obtain adequate protein and nutrients.[1] Mindful eating and the continued focus on the non-food related eating behaviors as outlined in Text Box 2, also play an important role in the long-term success of the bariatric patient.[11]

Table 4: A sample of a 1200-calorie maintenance diet (Adapted from Ref. 9).

Food Group	Servings/day	Food/Serving Size	Protein (g/serving)
Protein	8	1 oz. chicken, turkey breast, water packed tuna, salmon, shellfish, cod, tilapia, trout, egg, vegetarian meat substitute.	7
Dairy	2	1 cup skim milk or unsweetened soy milk, 1 oz low-fat cheese, 6 oz non-fat yogurt, ¼ cup fat-free ricotta or cottage cheese.	6–15
Whole Grains	4	1 slice whole wheat (high fiber) bread, $1/3$ cup brown rice, ½ cup cooked cereal, ¼ whole wheat bagel, 2 rice cakes.	3
Fruit	2	1 small apple or pear, ½ banana, ¾ cup berries, ½ cup canned fruit in juice, 15 grapes, 1 medium peach, ¼ cup dried fruit.	0
Vegetables	2	½ cup cooked or 1 cup raw: Asparagus, beets, broccoli, cabbage, cauliflower, cucumber, lettuce/leafy greens, zucchini.	2–3
Healthy Fats	2–3	1 teaspoon olive oil or canola oil, $1/8$ avocado, 1 teaspoon margarine, 2 tablespoons reduced fat salad dressing.	0

Recommendations for Macronutrient Intake

The macronutrient requirements after bariatric surgery are not yet clearly defined. Recommendations for the general population will be compared to current clinical macronutrient recommendations for WLS or data from observational studies of bariatric patients.

Protein

Adequate dietary protein is essential to prevent the breakdown of lean body mass during calorie restriction and to promote wound healing after surgery. The 2005 dietary reference intake (DRI) recommends the general adult population maintain a protein intake of approximately 50 to 60 g/d or 0.8 g/kg ideal body weight (IBW) for health.[8] The recommended goal for protein intake following bariatric surgery may be 60 to 80 g/d or 1.0 to 1.5 g/kg IBW.[2,5] While higher than the DRI, these recommendations are similar to those made for medically supervised protein sparing modified fasts and reduced calorie diets.[5]

Current protein recommendations appear to meet the needs of the majority of patients after RYGB, SG and AGB. In a small percentage of patients with malabsorptive operations such as the distal RYGB, protein malnutrition has been observed.[5,12] A higher protein intake of 1.5 g/kg IBW is recommended to help prevent loss of lean tissues.[13] However, due to the volume restrictions of surgery, it may be difficult for patients to achieve a higher protein intake without excluding other dietary macronutrients. A protein goal of 2.1 g/kg IBW is suggested for WLS patients requiring nutrition support.[14,15]

Fat

After surgery, fat in the diet should be limited to minimize calorie intake (fat contains 9 kcal/g, twice as much as protein or carbohydrates which contain 4 kcal/g). Some dietary fat is needed for the absorption of fat soluble vitamins, prostaglandin production and cellular structure. The minimum amount of fat necessary for metabolic needs of the general population is 20 to 25 g/d.[8] The quality of fat is also important and healthy sources of fat containing *n*-3 and *n*-6 fatty acids are essential.[9]

Dietary fat intake during the first year post bariatric surgery has been cited to range between 30% to 42% of energy intake.[9] It is recommended however, to keep fat intake in the lower end of the above range to insure adequate dietary protein and carbohydrate intake. In patients who are experiencing weight re-gain, a diet consisting of 20% of calories from dietary fat may be suggested.[1] This is consistent with the lower range of the DRI recommendation of 20% to 35% calories from fat for the general population.[8] To prevent dumping-like symptoms in RYGB patient's, fat should also be reduced, though data to the incidence of fat intolerance is limited.[9]

Carbohydrates

After WLS, carbohydrates should be limited, to allow for adequate protein intake. Sufficient amounts of carbohydrates are necessary to conserve protein. If carbohydrate intake is inadequate, it is possible to have loss of lean muscle mass through de-amination and release of carbon skeletons for energy.[16] Therefore, complex carbohydrates should be included in the diet after WLS to help maintain muscle mass. A daily minimal amount of carbohydrate is also required for normal cell activity, particularly red blood cells and neurons.

The minimum recommended dietary allowance for carbohydrates in the general adult population is 130 g/d.[8] It is observed that bariatric surgery patients frequently do not meet the minimum required for the general population. Studies have established that most bariatric patients are able to consume an average of 40% to 45% of calories from carbohydrate.[1,16] One study observed that 90 g/d of carbohydrate appeared adequate for RYGB patients six months post-op and intake of less than 130 g/d appeared adequate for patients one year or more post-surgery.[16] It is recommended that all patients avoid simple sugars and select complex carbohydrates and good sources of dietary fiber.

Micronutrient Requirements, Risk of Deficiencies and Laboratory Monitoring

An increased prevalence of micronutrient deficiencies, particularly of vitamin D, zinc, B-12, folate and iron have been observed in the morbidly obese.[14,17,18] Pre-operative assessment of micronutrient status is essential in order to correct deficiencies before surgery and avoid postoperative nutrition related complications.[17] After WLS, patients must take vitamin and mineral supplements to minimize the risk of deficiencies that may result from restricted intake, selecting foods with low nutrient density, or food intolerances.[1] Changes in the gastrointestinal physiology after RYGB and SG may alter nutrient absorption leading to newly developed deficiencies with a higher incidence observed following RYGB.[17,18] Vitamin deficiencies following AGB are less likely and in one prospective study were not observed after 7 years of follow-up even though inconsistent supplement use was noted.[19] Recommendations for vitamin and mineral supplement are outlined in Table 5.

All vitamin and mineral supplements should be approved by the bariatric dietitian and started before surgery. Patients must be made aware of the daily cost and the importance of committing to life-long supplementation.

Postoperative monitoring of nutrition-related laboratory values (Table 6) at 3 months, 6 months, 9 months and then annually or as needed, is required to detect deficiencies before they progress to functional impairments. Deficiencies, when identified, should be promptly treated following established institutional protocols.[2]

Patients with disease-specific nutritional needs, such as individuals with chronic kidney disease or on dialysis, may require specialized vitamin formulations and require modifications in the delivery of nutritional supplements.[20] Depending on the presence of co-morbid conditions additional laboratory monitoring may be needed.

Calcium

Elemental calcium citrate supplements providing between 1,200 to 1,500 mg/d should be recommended to prevent bone resorption and metabolic bone disease.[1] It has been suggested from a meta-analysis that the citrated form of calcium is better absorbed, when taken with and without food, than calcium carbonate by 22% to 27%.[21] For optimal absorption, patients should also be advised to take calcium in divided doses of ≤ 600 mg and to separate calcium

Table 5: Recommended Vitamin and Mineral Supplement use after WLS. (Adapted from Ref. 1 and 2)

Supplement	Dose	Required Daily Following		
		AGB	SG	RYGB
Multivitamin plus minerals	1 or 2 tablets per day dependent on the procedure	1	2	2
• Adult product				
• Must contain 100% DRI* for $\frac{2}{3}$ nutrients including thiamin, iron and folic acid.				
• Chewable or liquid products suggested for the first three months				
Calcium citrate	1,200 to 1,500 mg/d	yes	yes	yes
Vitamin D	3,000 International Units/d	yes	yes	yes
• Include vitamin D in multivitamin and calcium supplements				
• Add additional Vitamin D as needed				
Vitamin B-12 use one of the following routes, to maintain normal reference range		**	yes	yes
• Sublingually tablet or liquid drops	≥ 500 mcg/d			
• Subcutaneous or intramuscular injection	1,000 mcg once a month or			
• Oral tablet	1,000 to 3,000 mcg/3 to 6 months ≥ 350 mcg/d			
• Nasal spray	500 mcg once a week			
Iron	40 to 60 mg/d	**	yes	yes
• Include iron in multivitamin supplement				
• Add additional iron as needed				

* DRI — Dietary Reference Intake for Americans.

** AGB placement does not alter nutrient absorption additional supplementation beyond daily multivitamin may not be needed.

Table 6: Nutrition-related Laboratory Tests Monitored after Bariatric Surgery (Adapted from Ref 1).

Comprehensive metabolic panel

    Albumin

    Total Protein

    Electrolytes

    Glucose

    Bilirubin

Complete blood count with platelets

    Hemoglobin

    Hematocrit

    MCV

    MCH

Additional studies

    Glycosylated hemoglobin (Hemoglobin A1C)

    Iron including Total iron, Ferritin, TIBC

    Lipid Profile

    Liver Function Tests

    Vitamin D (25 (OH) vitamin D)

    Vitamin B-12, or Methylmalonic acid

    Folic Acid

    Thyroid Stimulating Hormone

    Intact PTH

    Thiamin

If *Failure to Thrive* include: Copper, Zinc and Selenium

supplements from multivitamins containing iron or iron supplements by 2 h.[2] The dose of supplemental calcium should be reduced as dietary sources of calcium-are included.[1]

Vitamin D

Vitamin D requirements are at least 3,000 IU/d from ergocalciferol (D2) or cholecalciferol (D3) and should be titrated to

maintain blood levels of >30 ng/mL 25-hydroxyvitamin D.[1]
Hyperparathyroidism and the prevalence of vitamin D deficiency
after bariatric surgery remains high.[22] Therefore, evaluation of
vitamin D status on an annual basis and bone density via DEXA
scan at 2 years is recommended to minimize bone loss and maintain bone health.[1]

Vitamin B-12

Patients who undergo a RYGB or SG require more vitamin B-12
than is found in a multivitamin. Bypassing or removing a large portion of the stomach during RYGB or SG causes a decreased
availability of intrinsic factor which is needed for B-12 absorption in
the terminal ileum. Deficiency may also be related to incomplete
digestion and release of vitamin B-12 from protein foods due to
decreased acid production in the pouch and sleeve. AGB patients
may not need additional B-12 supplementation since digestion and
absorption is not changed with band placement. Vitamin B-12 supplementation guidelines are outlined in Table 5. The best route to
prevent deficiency is not known. Patient preference and commitment to daily supplement use or monthly injections should be
evaluated.

Preoperative screening and treatment of vitamin B-12 deficiencies (< 200 pg/mL), including low-normal levels (200–400 pg/mL),
is recommended to prevent rapid onset of postoperative deficiency.[2]
Methylmalonic acid (MMA) is the preferred marker of B-12 status
since changes in MMA often precede low cobalamin levels. Evaluation
of serum B-12 may miss 20% to 35% of the deficiencies making it a
less reliable test.[23]

The incidence of postoperative vitamin B-12 deficiency has been
reported in approximately 35% of postoperative RYGB patients and
has been associated with megaloblastic anemia, and neurological
symptoms including paresthesia and permanent nerve damage.[2]
The onset of deficiency has been observed as early as six months

after RYGB but most often occurs more than one year postoperatively as liver stores become exhausted.[2]

Iron

The recommended iron intake from food and supplements is 45 to 60 mg/d.[1] Multivitamins containing iron are recommended following bariatric surgery. Many multivitamins contain 18 mg of iron per tablet which is the Recommended Dietary Allowance (RDA) for iron in women between 19 and 50 years of age.[24] The RDA for iron in adult men and women over the age of 51 years is 8 mg/d.[24] Iron, TIBC and ferritin, along with hemoglobin and hematocrit, should be routinely monitored in all bariatric patients. Menstruating women, patients with a history of iron deficiency, or a change in laboratory values may need additional oral iron supplementation from ferrous sulfate, fumerate or gluconate forms, to provide up to 150–200 mg elemental iron daily.[1] Iron deficiency is common after RYGB due to decreased absorptive area resulting from bypassing the duodenum and proximal jejunum as well as the reduced dietary intake of iron-rich foods. If RYGB patients require additional iron, enteric coated or extended release tablets should be avoided due to the decreased overall absorptive area and the potential for decreased (shortened) transit time. After SG, iron absorption may be reduced due to less hydrochloric acid secretion by the stomach.[17] For optimal absorption it is recommended iron be taken with either a vitamin C containing food or with a 250 mg vitamin C supplement.[25] Iron infusions may be required for patients with severe intolerance to oral products or refractory deficiency due to severe malabsorption.

Thiamin

Thiamin deficiency, while rare, can develop in patients with severe, intractable vomiting and decreased intake due to stomal stenosis following RYGB.[2] Deficiency can develop rapidly with a period of weeks or a few months and has been observed as early as 1 to 3 months after surgery. Early diagnosis of decreased serum thiamine is essential to prevent serious health problems. Symptoms of early deficiency include anorexia, weakness, parasthesias, edema and lower blood pressure and body temperature. Advanced deficiency can result in beri beri, cardiac failure, peripheral neuropathy and myelopathy, more so in the legs than arms and Wernicke's encephalopathy or Wernicke's–Korsakoff Syndrome.[26] Patients with rapid weight loss and persistent vomiting, or with neuropathy or encephalopathy, heart failure or alcohol abuse should be treated empirically treated with intravenous thiamin.[1] Since thiamin is needed for carbohydrate metabolism, the infusion of intravenous dextrose without thiamin in the postoperative bariatric patient can deplete body stores and cause an acute deficiency.[26]

Copper

Recommended vitamin and mineral supplement should contain 2 mg/d of copper. While routine screening for copper status is not indicated, copper deficiency has been reported following RYGB. Copper status should be evaluated in those bariatric patients with unexplained hematologic and neurologic symptoms since deficiency can result in persistent deficits.[22]

Diet-Related Gastrointestinal Complications

Following bariatric surgery gastrointestinal complaints may be common and can appear days, weeks or years after surgery. Unpleasant symptoms such as discomfort, vomiting and dumping syndrome may result from dysfunctional eating behaviors. Attention to suggested diet progression, appropriate food selection and eating habits usually can minimize these undesirable effects, which if left untreated may promote the intake of inappropriate and less nutrient dense foods. However, prompt medical attention may be required first if symptoms are severe or persistent.

Dehydration

Inadequate fluid intake, in the early postoperative period, may cause nausea, and result in dehydration. Vomiting and diarrhea may also contribute to dehydration. To manage fluid intake patients should be encouraged to take frequent sips of fluids thought out the day. While fluid needs vary from patient to patient a minimum goal of 48 oz should be encouraged.[4] Intravenous fluids may be required to hydrate patients who complain of persistent nausea and are unable to achieve fluid goals early after surgery.

Nausea and Vomiting

Nausea and vomiting has been reported to occur in more than 50% of patients undergoing restrictive procedures.[27] Periodic episodes of nausea and vomiting may be related to food intolerances, (Table 7: Foods and beverages likely to cause GI distress or weight gain), result from eating or drinking too quickly or too much, or not chewing foods well enough. The basic principles of how to drink and eat should be reinforced to help patients minimize the frequency of these episodes. Due to the reduced ability of the stomach to grind food, large pieces of food can cause nausea and vomiting.

Persistent vomiting in the early post-op period may lead to dehydration and thiamin depletion, and must be evaluated immediately.[26] Recurrent vomiting particularly in the first 2–3 months after surgery could be the result of a stricture of the gastrojejunostomy in the RYGB or a narrowing of the sleeve.[26] Patients may complain of inability to advance their diet or notice that they are only able to tolerate fluids. Treatment for a stricture is endoscopic balloon dilatation of the anastomosis or the sleeve. Several procedures may be required before the patient is able to tolerate diet advancement. During this period patients should be provided with dietary guidance to ensure nutritional goals are met and psychological or emotional support if a fear of eating has developed.

Occasionally patients will report self-induced vomiting[28] to relieve discomfort associated with eating too much or too fast. This

Table 7:   Foods and beverages likely to cause GI distress or weight gain.

Food/Nutrient	Recommendation/Rational
Sugar-containing foods, concentrated sweets.	Avoid foods with added sugar of more than 15 grams per serving. Sugar containing foods cause dumping syndrome (RYGB) and contribute to empty and excess calorie intake.
Fatty, fried foods.	Avoid high fat foods and frying foods. Caloric density of high fat foods may prevent weight loss. Frying makes food hard to digest and cause dumping like symptoms in RYGB.
Doughy bread products, rice, pasta.	Delay introduction. Avoid if intolerance causes "plugging" effect resulting in pain or nausea or vomiting.
Red meat, chicken.	Avoid tough and dry cuts of meat or poultry.
Nuts, fibrous vegetables, skin or peel of fruit or vegetables, citrus fruit membranes, popcorn.	Delay introduction. These foods may obstruct the stoma or gastric band opening.
Sugar alcohols.	Evaluate indivudual tolerance. Consume *in moderation* excess consumption can cause bloating, gas and loose bowel movements.
Acidic or spicy foods.	As tolerated.
Carbonated beverages.	Avoid, consumption results in abdominal pain and distention.
Sugar containing beverages.	Avoid drinks with added sugar; limit 100% fruit juice to 6 oz a day. Liquid calories can prevent weight loss. Sugar containing liquids can cause dumping syndrome.
Caffeine containing beverages.	Wean prior to surgery to avoid headaches associated with caffeine withdrawal. Usually avoided in early post-op diet. Reintroduce *in moderation*, when fluid intake consistently meets goals.
Alcohol	RYGB avoid due to impaired metabolism. AGB & SG avoid for 6 to 12 months, then *in moderation* due to caloric content of alcoholic beverages.

(Continued)

Table 7: (*Continued*)

Food/Nutrient	Recommendation/Rational
Lactose containing foods & beverages	If lactose intolerant avoid milk, other dairy products if severe. Choose lactose-free milk products or alternatives such as unsweetened soy or fortified almond milk. Select lactose-free protein supplements such as products with whey protein isolates or vegetable protein.

practice should be discouraged and appropriate eating practices and food selection should be reviewed.

Early Dumping Syndrome

Gastric dumping is an undesirable postoperative side effect seen after RYGB. Dumping is usually due to poor food and beverage choices and occurs as a result of rapid emptying of sugars or carbohydrates from the gastric pouch into the small intestine.[29] Also eating and drinking at the same time may cause rapid digestion of food resulting in increased intake and dumping-like symptoms following RYGB and SG.

Early dumping occurs 30 to 60 min postprandial and can last up to 60 min.[29] Symptoms include palpitations, fatigue, flushing, epigastric fullness, diarrhea, nausea, vomiting and abdominal cramps. Studies suggest that dumping occurs in approximately 50% to 71% of RYGB patients.[28] To prevent dumping, instruct patients to eliminate concentrated sweets and select foods with less than 15 g of sugar in a serving. It is also advised to avoid greasy, high-fat and fried foods, as well as separate drinking and eating by 30 min. The threat of dumping usually provides the negative reinforcement to help patients abide by the diet principles and stay away from calorie dense foods that can interfere with weight loss. Over time however, intestinal adaption may occur and the negative effects of eating foods with simple sugars and fat are blunted. Therefore appropriate low calorie food selection is a lifelong goal.

Late Stage Dumping and Postprandial Hypoglycemia

Late stage dumping, which is also known as postprandial hyperin-sulinemic hypoglycemia or reactive hypoglycemia, occurs 1 to 3 h after eating and usually presents 1 to 2 years after RYGB. The symptoms most frequently reported by patients are lightheadedness, diaphoresis, dizziness, fatigue, weakness or loss of consciousness.[30] The prevalence is unknown.[30] Postprandial hypoglycemia may results from an exaggerated release of insulin following a high carbohydrate meal.[30] Treatment includes initiating a strict low carbohydrate diet, eliminating simple sugars and eating well balanced small meals at regular intervals as well as separating eating and drinking.[31] If the response to dietary modification is inadequate, an alpha-glucosidase inhibitor can be added.[30] If symptoms persist, adjunctive treatment with somatostatin may be useful.[30]

Food Intolerances

Reports of food intolerance causing gastrointestinal distress, pain, nausea or vomiting vary considerably and are not experienced by all bariatric patients. The foods commonly cited to cause intolerance are dry, tough meat and poultry, sticky, doughy bread products or pasta, raw or stringy vegetables (Table 7: Foods and beverages likely to cause GI distress or weight gain).[4] These foods may not be easy to chew or digest through the narrow stoma, anastomosis or sleeve. Suggesting that only one new food is introduced at a time in the early postoperative period may help patients identify items causing discomfort. Repeated attempts to eat offending foods should be discouraged to prevent poor intake or dehydration. Development of intolerance to protein containing foods, specifically red meats, pork, or chicken, may eventually compromise protein intake.[13]

Lactose Intolerance

Lactose intolerance may be observed after surgery and is likely due to decreased production of the intestinal enzyme, lactase. Increased consumption of low fat dairy product may precipitate symptoms of lactose intolerance including flatulence, bloating, abdominal cramping and diarrhea. Lactose intolerant patients are instructed to choose lactose-free milk products or milk-alternatives, such as unsweetened soy or fortified almond milks and select lactose free protein supplements. Oral lactase tablets can be purchased over the counter and used with dairy products to prevent unpleasant side effects. The ingredient label on foods should be checked for hidden sources of lactose, such as dried milk solids, casein, caseinate, milk protein and whey protein concentrate.

Dysphagia to Solid Foods

Dysphagia particularly after AGB placements can be caused by eating too quickly, taking too big a mouthful, not chewing food adequately, eating food that is hard to chew to pureed consistency, or eating doughy foods. Following band placement some patient report symptoms of dysphagia early in the day with resolution of symptoms as the day progresses. Drinking a glass of warm liquid or water 30 min before breakfast may help to alleviate difficulty with solids. Recommending a liquid meal replacement or protein-containing beverage will help patients maintain appropriate nutrition and decrease anxiety associated with dysphagia.

Obstruction of the Outlet of the Pouch

Following AGB placement a bolus of food can obstruct the outlet of the pouch causing severe pain. Vomiting or regurgitation may relieve the obstruction. However, if symptoms persist and liquid, including saliva, is not tolerated, all fluid in the band should be removed to permit the food bolus to pass through the stoma. If deflating the band does not work, endoscopy may be required to remove the obstruction.

To prevent obstruction of the pouch patients should be instructed to slow the pace of eating taking 20–30 min per meal, to chew food to pureed consistency before swallowing and allow the food to pass across the band before the second bite is taken. Also patients should be instructed to avoid dry meats, dense protein, doughy starches and stringy fibrous vegetables which may block the gastric outlet.

Reflux and Reflux–like Symptoms

AGB patients may experience reflux-like symptoms if food is consumed quickly causing stacking above the pouch in the esophagus. To prevent discomfort it is important to instruct patients to eat slowly and chew food thoroughly to a mushy consistency. If the AGB is too tight, has slipped, or if the stomach is prolapsed above the band, symptoms of reflux may occur. Treatment in these instances may include removing the fluid from the band or another surgery to reposition the band may be required.

Sleeve gastrectomy patients often report gastroesophageal reflux symptoms in the early postoperative period. Over time, the incidence of reflux significantly decreases or can improve.[32] Foods causing symptoms should be avoided. Proton pump inhibitors may be used for three months postoperatively to minimize symptoms.

Constipation

Decreased food and fluid intake, the initial focus on high protein and low fiber food and the use of calcium and iron supplementation may cause constipation following bariatric surgery. Narcotic use for pain control will also slow bowel function after surgery. Fiber supplements can be added. Adequate fluid intake should accompany increased fiber consumption. Stool softeners and laxatives can also be recommended when indicated.

Malnutrition

Malnutrition or failure-to–thrive, following WLS is not common but may occur if dietary intake is chronically sub-optimal and dietary goals are not achieved.[2] Conditions or behaviors negatively impacting nutrition status after bariatric surgery include: alcohol or drug abuse, anorexia, depression, diarrhea, fear of regaining weight, food intolerance, limited resources for food and supplements and prolonged vomiting.

Nutrition Support of the Bariatric Patient

The implementation of parenteral or enteral nutrition should be considered in the high risk bariatric patient unable to tolerate oral nutrition for more than 3 to 7 days if critically ill, or 5 to 7 days with non-critical illness.[1] Nutrition support guidelines for the hospitalized patient with obesity, body mass index > 30, have been published by the American Society for Parenteral and Enteral Nutrition.[14] Hypocaloric (50% to 70% energy expenditure as determined by indirect calorimetry), high protein (2 to 2.5 g/kg IBW) feedings are encouraged in patients who do not have severe renal or hepatic dysfunction.[14] If indirect calorimetry is unavailable, energy requirements should be calculated using the most appropriate predictive equation.[14] In addition appropriate medical, psychological, and dietary treatments should be instituted, including identification and repletion of micronutrient deficiency states as per institution protocol.[14]

Routine and Long-term Follow-up

Follow-up with the bariatric team, including nutrition monitoring and dietary counseling by a registered dietitian, is suggested at two weeks, six weeks, three months and six months after surgery. Thereafter, patients should make appointments annually or follow-up more frequently, if needed, for other medical or nutritional indications.[1,2] RYGB patients who returned for all follow-up visits have greater long- term weight loss than those who did not return.[33] Unfortunately compliance with follow-up visits seems to decline over time with one study noting 90% of patients returning at two weeks, 54% at one year, 22% at two years and only 10% at three years.[28]

During follow-up visits the dietitian should assess fluid and protein intake, portion size, food texture and tolerance, frequency of eating, and use of vitamin and mineral supplements. Patient compliance with diet principles as well as readiness to advance diet should be discussed. Recent lab values should be reviewed and abnormalities corrected. Patients should be questioned about feelings of hunger and satiety and how they respond to these physiological cues. For the AGB patient an adjustment or fill, which is the process of adding fluid to the band over time to help limit food intake, should be based on the parameters noted in Table 8: Adjustable gastric band nutrition follow-up.[34]

Calorie intake

It has been demonstrated that over time calorie intake will increase after WLS.[35,36] In a study following RYGB patients, calorie intake was approximately 1,200 kcal/d at 20 weeks after surgery, and increased to 1,400 kcal/d by 92 weeks.[35] Individuals reporting high levels of dietary adherence had lost more weight.[35] A long term study of RYGB patients observed that calorie intake at 6 months after surgery was 1,500 kcal/d, and ten years later, calorie intake increased to 2,000 kcal/d.[36] Patients in this study regained approximately 10% of the maximum weight loss.[36]

Table 8: Adjustable gastric band nutrition follow-up.

Adjustment Schedule	Timeline	Nutrition Assessment
First adjustment	6 weeks post-op	• Assess tolerance to diet and eating behaviors.
On-going adjustments	Every 4 to 6 weeks as needed	Add fluid if: • Hunger reported between meals. • Appetite increased. • Larger portions are tolerated. • No weight loss or weight gain.
Criteria for fluid removal	As needed	Remove fluid if dietary changes do not resolve: • Persistent dysphasia. • Frequent regurgitation. • Maladaptive eating behaviors. • Development of a night cough. • Severe reflux or heartburn symptoms.

Successful weight loss is dependent on continuing calorie restriction. The dietitian should work with the patient at each follow-up visit to estimate the daily calorie needs, taking into account variables such as physical activity, weight loss progression, and protein intake.[9]

Weight Loss and Weight Maintenance

In the first 3 months after RYGB weight loss ranging between 40 and 90 lb may be observed due to very restricted calorie intake.[37] This translates into a loss of 0.5 to 1.0 lb per day[37] Weight loss is more gradual at 6 to 9 months with the goal being 1 to 2 lbs per week. After RYGB, maximum weight loss is achieved by 12 to 18 months and averages 61% excess body weight.[38] Weight loss following SG can be achieved in 1 to 2 years following surgery and is similar to the weight loss observed with the RYGB approximately 60% of excess body weight.[32,39] A more gradual weight loss is observed with the AGB with weight goals achieved after 2 to 3 years and averaging 48% of excess body weight.[38]

Weight loss alone should not be the only parameter used to define success following bariatric surgery. Resolution or improvement in comorbid conditions, improved sense of well-being and quality of life are also important factors to consider when evaluating surgical outcomes.[38]

Weight regain may occur after WLS. Weight lost from baseline at 10 years following surgery is 25% for RYGB and 14% for the AGB.[40] Factors commonly associated with inadequate weight loss or weight regain include binge eating disorder (BED), grazing or excessive snacking of calorie dense foods, maladaptive eating behaviors, psychological issues, or inadequately adjusted bands.[1]

Other important factors for successful weight loss and weight maintenance include exercise, support groups and self-monitoring. Becoming physically active after bariatric surgery is associated with better weight loss outcomes and mental health related quality of life.[41] A minimum of 150 min of moderate aerobic physical activity should be encouraged with a goal of 300 min per week. Strength training should also be incorporated 2 to 3 times per week.[1] Patients should also be encouraged to participate in ongoing support groups.[1] Regular self-weighing should be encouraged as a strategy for successful weight management.[42] The registered dietitian should also advise patients to keep an ongoing food and activity log for increased dietary compliance.

Conclusion

As nutrition experts registered dietitians must be active members of the multidisciplinary bariatric team. While WLS influences the volume of food consumed, dietary quality, compliance with supplement intake, eating behaviors and exercise patterns are important lifelong considerations for patients. The need for ongoing patient assessment and monitoring to prevent nutrient deficiencies and maximize long term weight loss and achieve positive health outcomes cannot be overemphasized.

References

1. AACE/TOS/ASMBS (2013) Clinical practice guidelines for the perioperative nutritional, metabolic, and nonsurgical support of the bariatric surgery patient. *Surg Obes Res Dis* **9**: 159–191.
2. Aills L, Blankenship J, Buffington C, Furtado M, Parrott J. (2008) ASMBS Allied Health Nutrition guidelines for the surgical weight loss patient. *Surg Obes Relat Dis* **4**(5 suppl): S73–S108.
3. Buzby, KM (2014) Bariatric Surgery. In: Matarese LE, Mullin CE, Raymond JL (eds) The health professionals guide to gastrointestinal nutrition, pp 182–202 Academy of Nutrition and Dietetics.
4. Parks E. (2006) Nutritional management of patients after bariatric surgery. *Am J Med Sci* **331**(4): 207–213.
5. Blankenship J, Wolfe B. (2006) Nutrition and Roux-en-Y Gastric Bypass. In: Sugerman HJ, Nguyen NT (eds.), *Management of morbid obesity*, pp. 75–89. Taylor & Francis, New York.
6. Castellanos VH, Litchford MD, Campbell WW. (2006) Modular protein supplements and their application to long-term care. *Nutr clin pract* **21**: 485–504.

7. Faria SL, Faria OP, Buffington C, de Almeida Cardeal M, Ito MK. (2011) Dietary protein intake and bariatric surgery patients: A review. *Obes Surg* **21**: 1798–1805.

8. National Academy of Sciences, Institute of Medicine. Food and Nutrition Board. (2002/2005) *Dietary reference intakes for energy, carbohydrate, fiber, fat, fatty acids, cholesterol, protein, and amino acids (macronutrients).* Retrieved from https://fnic.nal.usda.gov/dietary-guidance/dri-nutrient-reports/energy-carbohydrate-fiber-fat-fatty-acids-cholesterol-protein#overlay-context=dietary-guidance/dietary-reference-intakes/dri-reports. Accessed January 2014.

9. Moizé VL, Pi-Sunyer X, Mochari H, Vidal J. (2010) Nutritional pyramid for post-gastric bypass patients. *Obes Surg* **20**: 1133–1141.

10. Swenson BR, Schulman AS, Edwards MJ, Gross MP, Hedrick TL, Weltman AL, *et al.* (2007) The effect of a low-carbohydrate, high-protein diet on post laparoscopic gastric bypass weight loss: A prospective randomized trial. *J Surg Res* **142**: 308–313.

11. Piechota, T. (2012) *The Complete Counseling Kit for Weight Loss Surgery.* Academy of Nutrition and Dietetics.

12. Brolin RE, LaMarca LB, Kenler HA, Cody KP. (2002) Malabsoptive gastric bypass in patients with super obesity. *J Gastrointest Surg* **6**: 195–203.

13. Moizé V, Geliebter A, Gluck ME, Yahav E, Lorence M, Colarusso T, *et al.* (2003) Obese patients have inadequate protein intake related to protein intolerance up to 1 year following roux-en-Y gastric bypass. *Obes Surg* **13**: 23–28.

14. Choban P, Dickerson R, Malone A, *et al.* (2013) A.S.P.E.N. clinical guidelines. Nutrition support of hospitalized patients with obesity. *J Parente Enteral Nutr* **37**: 714–744.

15. Schinkel ER, Pettine SM Adams E, Harris M. (2006) Impact of varying levels of protein intake on protein status indicators after gastric bypass in patients with multiple complications requiring nutrition support. *Obes Surg* **16**: 24–30.

16. Faria SL, Faria OP, Cardeal MA *et al.* (2013) Recommended levels of carbohydrate after bariatric surgery. *Bariatric Times* **10**(3): 16–21.

17. Damms-Machado A, Friedrich A, Kramer KM *et al.* (2012) Pre- and postoperative nutritional deficiencies in obese patients undergoing laparoscopic sleeve gastrectomy. *Obes Surg* **22**: 881–889.

18. Gehrer S, Kern B, Peters T, Christoffel-Courtin C, Peterli R. (2010) Fewer nutrient deficiencies after laparoscopic sleeve gastrectomy

(LSG) than after laparoscopic roux-y-gastric bypass (LRYGB) — a prospective study. *Obes Surg* **20**: 447–453.

19. Schouten R, Wiryasaputra DC, van Dielen FMH, van Gemert WG, Greve JWM. (2010) Long-term results of bariatric restrictive procedures: a prospective study. *Obes Surg* **20**: 1617–1626.
20. Lightner AL, Lau J, Obayashi P, Birge K, Melcher ML. (2011) Potential nutritional conflicts in bariatric and renal transplant patients. *Obes Surg* **12**: 1965–1970.
21. Sakhaee K, Bhuket T, Adams-Huet B, Rao DS. (1999) Meta-analysis of calcium bioavailability: A comparison of calcium citrate with calcium carbonate. *Am J Ther* **6**: 313–321.
22. Saltzman E and Karl JP. (2013) Nutrient deficiencies after gastric bypass surgery. *Ann Rev Nutr* **33**: 19.1–19.21.
23. Carmel R, Green R, Rosenblatt DS, Watkins D. (2003) Update on cobalamin, folate, and homocysteine. *Am Soc Hematol Educ Progrm* 62–81.
24. NIH Office of Dietary Supplements. Iron dietary supplement fact sheet. http://ods.od.nih.gov/factsheets/Iron-HealthProfessional. Accessed 19 February 2014.
25. Rhode BM, Shustik C, Christou NV, Mac Lean LD. (1999) Iron absorption and therapy after gastric bypass. *Obes Surg.* **9**: 17–21.
26. Aasheim, ET. (2008) Wernicke encephalopathy after bariatric surgery: A systemic review. *Ann Surg.* **248**: 714–720.
27. McMahon MM, Sarr MG, Clark MM, *et al.* (2006) Clinical management after bariatric surgery: Value of a multidisciplinary approach. *Mayo Clin Proc* **81**(10 Suppl): S34–S45.
28. Wardé-Kamar J, Rogers M, Flancbaum L, Laferrère B. (2004) Calorie intake and meal patterns up to 4 years after roux-en-Y gastric bypass surgery. *Obes Surg* **14**: 1070–1079.
29. ASMBS Public/Professional Education Committee. (2008) *Bariatric Surgery: Postoperative Concerns.* Retrieved from http://asmbs.org/wp/uploads/2014/05/bariatric_surgery_postoperative_concerns1.pdf
30. Kellogg TA, Bantle JP, Leslie DB, Redmond JB, Slusarek B, Swan T, *et al.* (2008) Postgastric bypass hyperinsulinemic hypoglycemia syndrome: Characterization and response to a modified diet. *Surg Obes Relat Dis.* **4**: 492–499.
31. Tack J, Arts J, Caenepeel P, De Wulf D, Bisschops R. (2009) Pathophysiology, diagnosis and management of postoperative dumping syndrome. *Nat Rev Gastroenterol Hepatol* **6**: 583–590.

32. Snyder-Marlow G, Taylor D, Lenhard J. (2010) Nutrition care for patients undergoing laparoscopic sleeve gastrectomy for weight loss. *J Am Diet Assoc.* **110**: 600–607.
33. Gould JC, Beverstein G, Reinhardt S, Garren MJ. (2007) Impact of routine and long-term follow-up on weight loss after laparoscopic gastric bypass. *Surg Obes Relat Dis* **3**: 627–630.
34. Shen R, Dugay G, Rajaram K, Cabrera I, Siegel N, Ren C. (2004) Impact of patient follow-up on weight loss after bariatric surgery. *Obes Surg* **14**: 514–519.
35. Sarwer DB, Wadden TA, Moore RH, Baker AW, Gibbons LM, Raper SE, *et al.* (2008) Preoperative eating behaviors, postoperative dietary adherence and weight loss following gastric bypass surgery. *Surg Obes Relat Dis* **4**(5): 640–646.
36. Sjöström L, Lindroos AK, Peltonen M *et al.* (2004) Lifestyle, diabetes, and cardiovascular risk factors 10 years after bariatric surgery. *N Engl J Med* **351**: 2683–2693.
37. AACE/TOS/ASMBS. (2009) Medical guidelines for clinical practice for the perioperative nutritional, metabolic, and nonsurgical support of the bariatric surgery patient. *Obestiy.* **17**(supple 1) S1–S69.
38. Buchwald H, Avidor Y, Braunwald E, Jensen MD, Pories W, Fahrbach K, Schoelles K. (2004) Bariatric Surgery: A systematic review and meta-analysis. *JAMA* **292**: 1724–1737.
39. Nocca D, Krawczykowsky D, Bomans B, *et al.* (2008) A prospective multicenter study of 163 sleeve gastrectomies: Results at 1 and 2 years. *Obes Surg* **18**: 560–565.
40. Sjöström L, Narbro K, Sjöström CD, *et al.* (2007) Effects of bariatric surgery on mortality in Swedish obese subjects. *N Engl J Med* **357**(8): 741–752.
41. Bond DS, Phelan S, Wolfe LG, Evans RK, Meador JG, Kellum JM, *et al.* (2009) Becoming physically active after bariatric surgery is associated with improved weight loss and health-related quality of life. *Obesity* **17**(1): 78–83.
42. Wing RR, Tate DF, Gorin AA, Raynor HA, Fava JL. (2006) A self-regulation program for maintenance of weight loss. *N Engl J Med* **355**(15): 1563–1571.

Chapter 10

Metabolic Impact of Bariatric Surgery

Aileen A. Murphy[*,‡] and Kevin M. Reavis[†,§]

*West Coast Surgical Associates, Walnut Creek, CA, USA
†The Oregon Clinic, Portland, OR, USA
‡aamurphy.do@gmail.com
§kreavis@orclinic.com

Background

Much attention in the field of bariatric surgery has been paid to outcomes regarding weight loss. Obesity however, adversely affects countless metabolic processes in the human body and bariatric surgery has been shown to effect positive outcomes in many of them. The most notable metabolic disorders treated with bariatric surgery include diabetes, hypertension, dyslipidemia, non-alcoholic steatohepatitis (NASH), metabolic syndrome (a combination of several metabolic endocrinopathies), gastrointestinal hormone imbalance, nesidioblastosis, immunosuppression and fertility disorders. There are multiple bariatric surgical procedures in the surgeon's armamentarium including purely restrictive procedures such as adjustable gastric banding and sleeve gastrectomy as well as those adding a diverting component to the procedure such as Roux-en-Y gastric bypass and biliopancreatic diversion (BPD) with or without duodenal switch (DS). Each of these varies in terms of resolution of metabolic disorders, yet all have positive roles that will be addressed in this chapter.

According to the Centers for Disease Control and Prevention National Center for Health Statistics over 35% of the adults in the United States are obese with a body mass index (BMI) greater than 30 kg/m^2. While obesity is a preventable disease, the incidence has doubled around the world since 1980 according to the World Health Organization (WHO). Patients with obesity suffer from multiple medical problems as a complication of excess weight gain, contributing to over 400,000 deaths in the United States annually. These patients often have diabetes, hypertension, or metabolic syndrome, which includes insulin resistance, hypertension and dyslipidemia. While many commonly have sleep apnea, back and joint pain and depression, they may also endure fertility complications, fatty liver disease and hormone imbalance.

Bariatric surgical procedures commonly performed, including adjustable band, sleeve gastrectomy, Roux-en-Y bypass and BPD, not only results in excess weight loss, but also resolution of the co-morbidities associated with obesity, specifically diabetes, hypertension and sleep apnea (Fig. 1). The metabolic changes that occur after bariatric surgery are still unclear and appear to be due to hormonal changes in the GI tract and not just secondary to weight loss.

Metabolic Comorbidities due to Obesity

Roughly one-third of the United States population is obese, with Pima Indians, Polynesians, African Americans and Latino Americans at the highest risk. Although metabolic comorbidities associated with obesity are not identically distributed amongst these patients, there are recognizable patterns with greater predictability as the severity of obesity increases. Impaired glucose tolerance leading to Type 2 Diabetes Mellitus (T2DM) typically manifests after excess weight gain, so it is common that a strict low calorie diet leads to improved glucose intolerance. Unfortunately a strict diet, exercise regimen, and the addition of insulin have proven to be ineffective in controlling and resolving diabetes in the morbidly obese population; the hormonal effect of incretin on insulin resistance is readily apparent in the obese patient population. Incretin hormones are endocrine

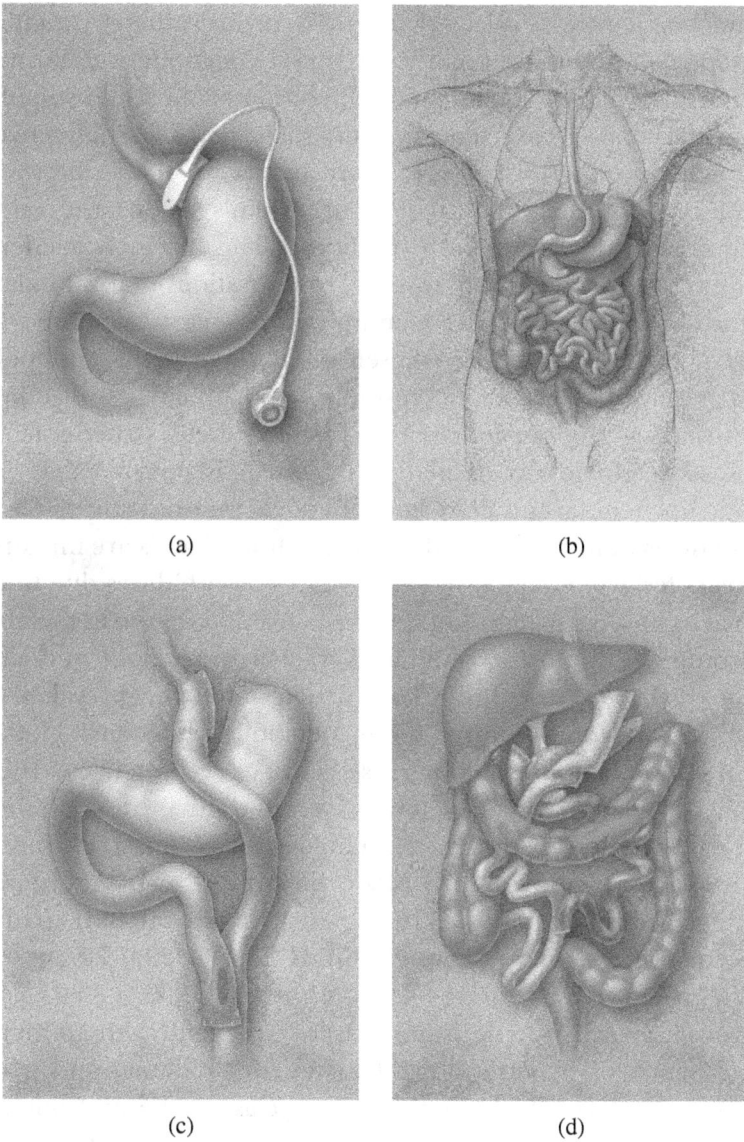

Figure 1 (A) Adjustable Gastric Band (B) Sleeve Gastrectomy (C) Gastric Bypass (D) Biliopancreatic Diversion.

insulinotropic factors released from the gut in response to glucose ingestion. Glucagon-like peptide-1 (GLP-1) is a gut-derived hormone that normally increases after an orally consumed meal and stimulates pancreatic beta-cells to release insulin which facilitates euglycemia.[1-4] Although, insulin resistance is characteristic of both obesity and T2DM, it is not established that all of insulin's actions are compromised in individuals with both conditions. The antilipolytic effect of insulin requires much lower insulin concentrations than stimulation of glucose transport. Hence, even in insulin-resistant states in which glucose transport is impaired, sensitivity to insulin's antilipolytic effect is relatively preserved, resulting in maintenance of adipose stores making the challenges that obese diabetic patients face in terms of weight loss particularly difficult. It is possible that while hepatic lipogenesis and lipid storage are excessive in adipose tissue, other effects of insulin related to glucose homeostasis are impaired.[5]

Diabetes, when combined with other comorbidities due to obesity makes up a particularly dangerous condition known as metabolic syndrome. Nguyen *et al.* evaluated 13,745 overweight and obese persons between 1999 and 2004 to determine the prevalence of metabolic syndrome amongst them. Metabolic syndrome includes at least three of the following: Increased waist circumference (>102 cm in men, >88 cm in women), elevated serum triglycerides ($\geq$150 mg/dL), low high-density lipoprotein cholesterol (<40 mg/dL in men, <50 mg/dL in women), high blood pressure ($\geq$130/$\geq$85 mm Hg) and high serum glucose ($\geq$110 mg/dL). Based on BMI, patients were categorized into overweight (BMI 25.0 to 29.9 kg/m^2) and obesity classes 1 (BMI 30.0 to 34.9 kg/m^2), 2 (BMI 35 to 39.9 kg/m^2) and 3 (>40 mg/kg^2). The findings were consistent with an increasing presence of hypertension, diabetes, dyslipidemia and overall metabolic syndrome with each increasing class of obesity. Compared to normal weight individuals, three times as many patients with class 3 obesity suffered from metabolic syndrome. Similar findings were noted regarding hypertension, diabetes and dyslipidemia to varying degrees.[6] Increased levels of obesity are accompanied by more comorbid conditions which result in greater challenges in the medical management of this subset of patients.

The hormonal and local effects of adipose tissue in obesity continue to evolve as adipokines play a role in insulin resistance. The expression of TNF-α by adipose tissue was first described in the mid-1990s and since then, many adipokines have been described in the pathogenesis of the chronic inflammation and insulin resistance associated with obesity. The adipokines implicated in the metabolic changes in obesity include leptin and adiponectin and the cytokines responsible for chronic inflammation include TNF-α, IL-6, and macrophages.[7]

Effects of Bariatric Surgery on Metabolism

Bariatric surgery is the most effective treatment for medically refractory morbid obesity and its related comorbidities. Pories *et al.* noted as early as 1995, that gastric bypass provided long-term control of non-insulin-dependent diabetes mellitus (NIDDM). After a 14-year follow-up, 121 of 146 patients (82.9%) with NIDDM and 150 of 152 patients (98.7%) with glucose impairment maintained normal levels of plasma glucose, glycosylated hemoglobin and insulin. These effects appeared to be due primarily to a reduction in caloric intake. In addition to the control of weight and NIDDM, gastric bypass also resolved a number of other comorbidities of obesity, including hypertension, sleep apnea, cardiopulmonary failure, arthritis and infertility.[8] The GLP-1 response to a meal was still elevated 10 years after gastric bypass, suggesting the durability of the procedure on glucose tolerance.[9] Schauer *et al.* evaluated 150 patients with uncontrolled diabetes and randomized them to medical therapy alone vs medical therapy plus bariatric surgery (Roux-en-Y bastric bypass or sleeve gastrectomy). Glycemic control improved in all groups, with 3–4 fold increase in medical therapy plus bariatric surgery compared to medical therapy alone, with a greater difference in weight loss and decrease in lipid lowering medications.[10] Adams *et al.* retrospectively reviewed 9,949 gastric bypass patients and 9,628 severely obese control subjects during a mean follow-up of 7.1 years. Adjusted long-term mortality from any cause in the surgery group decreased by 40%, as compared with that in the control group (37.6 vs 57.1

deaths per 10,000 person-years, $P < 0.001$); cause-specific mortality in the surgery group decreased by 56% for coronary artery disease (2.6 vs 5.9 per 10,000 person-years, $P = 0.006$), by 92% for diabetes (0.4 vs 3.4 per 10,000 person-years, $P = 0.005$), and by 60% for cancer (5.5 vs 13.3 per 10,000 person-years, $P < 0.001$). Long-term total mortality after gastric bypass surgery was significantly reduced, particularlydeaths from diabetes, heart disease, and cancer.[11] The Swedish Obese subjects study showed similar results in overall reduction in mortality after bariatric surgery after 10 year follow-up. In this study Sjöström *et al.* evaluated 4,047 morbidly obese individuals, 2,010 underwent bariatric surgery (376 underwent non-adjustable or adjustable gastric banding, 1,369 underwent vertical banded gastroplasty, the precursor of adjustable gastric banding, and 265 underwent gastric bypass) while 2,037 were treated medically. The mean weight change in the medically treated group was less than 2%, 15 years following enrollment in the study. Highest weight loss results were observed in the surgical group of patients after one to two years. Patients undergoing gastric bypass had a mean of 32% weight loss while those undergoing vertical banded gastroplasty lost a mean of 25% and those with banding lost a mean of 20%. Ten years following treatment weight loss from baseline had stabilized at 25%, 16% and 14% respectively. The unadjusted overall hazard ratio was 0.76 in the surgery group ($P = 0.04$), as compared to the control group and the hazard ratio adjusted for sex, age and risk factors was 0.71 ($P = 0.01$).[12]

When assessing metabolic syndrome in similarly obese patients, the dangers of this condition become even more apparent. Among patients in the same obesity class, those suffering with metabolic syndrome are at greater health risk than those without metabolic syndrome. Varela *et al.* evaluated the in-hospital outcomes of 20,242 patients undergoing bariatric surgery. Obese patients who suffered with metabolic syndrome were compared with those who did not have the syndrome. Although mortality between the two groups was similar and well-below 0.1%, patients with metabolic syndrome were nearly 50% more likely (8.6% vs 5.8%) to suffer a postoperative complication compared to their counterparts without metabolic syndrome. Hispanic males were noted to be at greatest risk and due to its short term safety profile and 92% efficacy in halting metabolic syndrome, laparoscopic adjustable gastric banding (LAGB) was seen as the best short term surgical treatment for metabolic syndrome in these patients.[13]

Fortunately, multiple comorbidities associated with obesity are treated effectively with bariatric surgery. Hinojosa *et al.* followed 95 obese patients being treated for hypertension with Roux-en-Y gastric bypass and found the majority had either complete resolution (46%) or significant improvement (additional 19%) in their comorbid state. Treatability of hypertension was noted to be inversely related to the length of time each patient had the disorder prior to surgery.[14]

Other metabolic disorders such as dyslipidemia are also effectively addressed with bariatric surgery. Vila *et al.*[15] evaluated 67 non-diabetic patients before and one year following BPD and Zambon *et al.*[16] evaluated 15 non-diabetic patients before and one year following LAGB. In both studies significant reductions in triglyceride and low density lipoprotein (LDL) levels were observed through follow-up. This was accompanied in both studies with significant increases in high density lipoprotein levels. Overall atherogenic LDL profiles were improved resulting in potentially improved cardiac risk stratification in these patients.

The effects of bariatric surgery on lipid metabolism are not limited to serum lipid stores. The effects of surgery are also appreciated in the abdominal viscera and subcutaneous regions. Heath *et al.* evaluated 18 female patients who underwent magnetic resonance imaging before as well as 3 and 12 months after LAGB to quantify abdominal subcutaneous and visceral adipose tissue areas as well as liver fat content. Following surgery, significant adipose tissue loss was noted in both visceral and subcutaneous regions with greater loss noted in abdominal viscera. Significant adipose tissue reduction of the liver was only observed in surgical patients in whom a pre-operative diagnosis of hepatic steatosis existed.[17] Similarly de Andrade *et al.* found that upon histological and ultrasonic inspection, Non-alcoholic fatty liver disease (NAFLD) was significantly impacted following bariatric surgery.

In this study, 40 patients agreed to undergo intraoperative liver biopsy with ultrasound and serum markers measured during follow-up carried out to a mean of 21 months. All 40 patients had NAFLD on histological evaluation. Upon follow-up completion only 1 of 40 still met criteria for NAFLD. Pre-operatively all 40 patients met criteria for Fatty Liver index with scores >60. At completion of follow-up, only 27.5% still had scores >60. These findings were also reflected in anthropomorphic measurements. Although all patients had waist circumferences meeting criteria for metabolic syndrome (>102 cm, male; and >88 cm, female) before the study, only 52% had waist circumferences of this magnitude at completion of follow-up.[18]

Hyperinsulinemic hypoglycemia has been reported following Roux-en-Y gastric bypass in some patients. This is a rare phenomenon and the etiology, physiology and exact incidence are still being determined. Due to islet cell hyperplasia (nesidioblastosis) being postulated as the likely source for this condition, distal or subtotal pancreatectomy has been used in several cases to treat the disorder. Z'graggen *et al.* found that a more simple approach involving the restoration of appropriate levels of gastric restriction may be all that is necessary to reverse this debilitating condition. In their study, 12 patients suffering from post-bypass hyperinsulinemic hypoglycemia were treated with placement of a silastic band ($n = 4$) or adjustable gastric band ($n = 8$) around the dilated gastric pouch and followed for a median of seven months. Five of the 12 patients underwent open surgery and pancreatic biopsies were obtained. Two of the five had histological evidence of nesidioblastosis as the etiology for the hypoglycemic episodes, whereas three were due to other causes. At the completion of follow-up, hypoglycemic episodes had resolved in 9 of the 12 patients with banding alone and three required treatment with additional partial pancreatectomy to achieve resolution of the condition.[19]

Leptin and ghrelin, opposing appetite hormones, have recently garnered significant interest both from the surgical and pharmaceutical communities as potential targets to impact obesity and the metabolic sequelae that accompany it. Leptin, produced in adipose tissue serves to inhibit appetite, while ghrelin, produced in the gastric fundic mucosa serves as an appetite stimulus. In obese patients leptin is usually higher and ghrelin is lower than in normal subjects. Following weight loss, conventional wisdom leads us to anticipate drops in leptin and increases in ghrelin to levels above those in normal individuals. With surgically induced weight loss, this phenomenon is not the case. Shak *et al.* followed 24 patients under-going adjustable gastric banding over a 12 month period. Median excess body weight loss was 45.7%. Leptin levels dropped by 65% and ghrelin levels remained fairly stable.[20] In a similar 12 month follow-up study evaluating the effects of gastric bypass, Pardina *et al.* analyzed the hormonal changes in 34 patients. Preoperatively leptin levels were 147% of normal and ghrelin levels were 46% below normal. One year following surgery, leptin levels dropped by 75% and ghrelin levels increased by 78% however, both hormone levels settled below that of normal subjects at the completion of follow-up.[21]

In addition to the effects of bariatric surgery on metabolic syndrome, appetite and gastrointestinal physiology, improvements in immunocompetency and fertility have also been observed. Gagné *et al.* investigated 49 patients, nearly all of whom underwent laparoscopic Roux-en-Y gastric bypass, who had pre-operatively required immunosuppressive medication to treat disorders including asthma, osteoarthritis, psoriasis, myasthenia gravis and rheumatoid arthritis. At median follow-up of 18 months 51% of patients were completely free of immunosuppressive medication requirements and overall 66%–100% of patients had either significant reductions or complete discontinuation of their medications for these various conditions.[22] Rochester *et al.* evaluated nine morbidly obese women (mean BMI 47.3) who underwent bariatric surgery and lost >25% of their initial body weight by the sixth postoperative month. Preoperatively, these women were noted to have deficient luteal luteinizing hormone and pregnanediolglucuronide excretion compared with normal-weight women. Six months following surgery, whole-cycle luteinizing hormone increased from 168.8 +/− 24.2 to 292.1 +/− 79.6 mIU/mg Creatinine and luteal pregnanediolglucuronide more than doubled from 32.8 to 73.7 μg/mg Creatinine.[23]

Bariatric surgery in the setting of polycystic ovarian syndrome (PCOS) has varied results. Escobar-Morreale *et al.* evaluated premenopausal morbidly obese women with and without PCOS after BPD or gastric bypass. All PCOS patients had recovery of regular ovulatory cycles, improvement in hirsutism, and nearly normal serum androgen levels and the diagnosis of PCOS could no longer be sustained in these patients after bariatric surgery.[24] Eid *et al.* had similar results in the 24 women with PCOS who had undergone gastric bypass, with improvement in hirsutism.[25] In the rat model for PCOS and chronic dihydrotestotsterone, sleeve gastrectomy has shown loss of weight and body fat, without improvement of glucose tolerance or recovery of estrous ovulation.[26]

The impact on female fertility in obese patients of these findings is still being determined, underscoring the complexity of reproductive endocrinology and the role surgery may play in bringing the possibility of fertility to morbidly obese women for whom reproduction can be a tremendously frustrating challenge.

Relative Impact of Various Bariatric Surgeries

The therapeutic impact on metabolic comorbidities appears to correlate directly with the technical complexity of the operative interventions and associated excess weight loss. LAGB is a purely restrictive procedure that requires multiple adjustments to the band volume before weight loss goals are achieved. LAGB results in more excess weight loss than medical therapy alone and thus has modest effects on diabetes, hypertension, dyslipidemia, GERD, PCOS and NASH. Laparoscopic sleeve gastrectomy is also a purely restrictive procedure, but results in more excess weight loss and thus has a larger improvement on those medical ailments, with the exception of GERD and PCOS. Gastric bypass has better resolution of GERD and PCOS; and with the exception of GERD, BPD/DS is the most impactful in terms of comorbidity treatment and resolution in the morbidly obese population (Table 1).

Although bariatric surgery has had a tremendous impact in weight reduction and amelioration of diabetes and metabolic

Table 1   Resolution of co-morbidities in obesity after bariatric surgery.

	Medical	Gastric Band	Sleeve Gastrectomy	Gastric Bypass	BPD/DS
Diabetes	+	++	+++	+++	++++
Hypertension	+	++	+++	+++	++++
Dyslipidemia	+	++	+++	+++	++++
GERD	+	+/−	+/−	+++	++
PCOS	+	++	+/−	+++	+++
NASH	+	+	++	+++	+++

syndrome in morbidly obese patients opting for surgery, the greatest contributions of this emerging discipline are still being discovered. Of the areas of bariatric research being addressed, the resolution of comorbid metabolic endocrinopathies, serves as one that has only recently started to realize its potential. Emerging translational research in this arena is now uniting multiple medical disciplines in the pursuit of someday resolving this plague of the human condition.

References

1. Holst JJ. (1994) Glucagon-like peptide 1: A newly discovered gastrointestinal hormone. *Gastroenterol* **107**: 1848–1855.
2. Tanizawa Y, Riggs AC, Elbein SC *et al.* (1994) Human glucagon-like peptide-I receptor gene in NIDDM. *Diabetes* **43**: 752–757.
3. Gutniak M, Orskov C, Holst JJ *et al.* (1992) Antidiabetogenic effect of glucagon-like peptide- 1 (7–36) in normal subjects and patients with diabetes mellitus. *N Engl J Med* **326**: 1316–1322.
4. Creutzfeldt W, Nauck M. (1992) Gut hormones and diabetes mellitus. *Diabetes Metab Rev* **8**: 149–177.
5. Kahn BB and Flier JS. (2000) Obesity and insulin resistance. *J Clin Invest* **106**(4): 473–481.
6. Nguyen NT, Magno CP, Lane KT, Hinojosa MW, Lane JS. (2008) Association of hypertension, diabetes, dyslipidemia, and metabolic syndrome with obesity: Findings from the National Health and Nutrition Examination Survey, 1999 to 2004. *J Am Coll Surg* **207**(6): 928–934.

7. Kern PA. (1997) Potential role of TNFα and lipoprotein lipase as candidate genes for obesity. *J Nutr* **127**(9): 19175–19225.

8. Pories WJ, Swanson MS, MacDonald KG, Long SB, Morris PG, Brown BM, Barakat HA, deRamon RA, Israel G, Dolezal JM, Dohm L. (1995) Who would have thought it? An operation proves to be the most effective therapy for adult-onset Diabetes Mellitus. *Ann Surg* **222**(3): 339–352.

9. Dar MS, Chapman WH, Drake AJ, O'Brien K, Tanenberg RJ, Dohm GL, Pories WJ. (2012) GLP-1 response to a mixed meal: What happens 10 years after Roux-en-Y gastric bypass (RYGB)? *Obes Surg* online. 15 March 2012.

10. Schauer PR, Kashyap SR, Wolski K, Brethauer SA, Kirwan JP, Pothier CE, Thomas S, Abood B, Nissen SE, Bhatt DL. (2012) Bariatric surgery versus intensive medical therapy in obese patients with Diabetes. *N Engl J Med* **366**: 1567–1576.

11. Adams TD, Gress RE, Smith SC, Halverson RC, Simper SC, Rosamond WD, LaMonte MJ, Stroup AM, Hunt SC. Long-term mortality after gastric bypass surgery. *N Engl J Med* **357**: 753–761.

12. Sjöström L, Narbro K, Sjöström CD, Karason K, Larsson B, Wedel H, Lystig T, Sullivan M, Bouchard C, Carlsson B, Bengtsson C, Dahlgren S, Gummesson A, Jacobson P, Karlsson J, Lindroos AK, Lönroth H, Näslund I, Olbers T, Stenlöf K, Torgerson J, Ågren G Carlsson LMS. (2007) Effects of bariatric surgery on mortality in Swedish obese subjects. *N Engl J Med* **357**: 741–752.

13. Varela JE, Hinojosa MW, Nguyen NT. (2008) Bariatric surgery outcomes in morbidly obese with the metabolic syndrome at US academic centers. *Obes Surg* **18**(10): 1273–1277.

14. Hinojosa MW, Varela JE, Smith BR, Che F, Nguyen NT. (2009) Resolution of systemic hypertension after laparoscopic gastric bypass. *J Gastrointest Surg* **13**(4): 793–797.

15. Vila M, Ruíz O, Belmonte M *et al.* (2009) Changes in lipid profile and insulin resistance in obese patients after Scopinarobiliopancreatic diversion. *Obes Surg* **19**(3): 299–306.

16. Zambon S, Romanato G, Sartore G *et al.* (2009) Bariatric surgery improves atherogenic LDL profile by triglyceride reduction. *Obes Surg* **19**(2): 190–195.

17. Heath ML, Kow L, Slavotinek JP, Valentine R, Toouli J, Thompson CH. (2009) Abdominal adiposity and liver fat content 3 and 12 months after gastric banding surgery. *Metabol* **58**(6): 753–758.

18. de Andrade AR, Cotrim HP, Alves E *et al.* (2008) Nonalcoholic fatty liver disease in severely obese individuals: The influence of bariatric surgery. *Ann Hepatol* **7**(4): 364–368.

19. Z'graggen K, Guweidhi A, Steffen R *et al.* (2008) Severe recurrent hypoglycemia after gastric bypass surgery. *Obes Surg* **18**(8): 981–988.

20. Shak JR, Roper J, Perez-Perez GI *et al.* The effect of laparoscopic gastric banding surgery on plasma levels of appetite-control, insulinotropic, and digestive hormones. *Obes Surg* **18**(9): 1089–1096.

21. Pardina E, López-Tejero MD, Llamas R *et al.* (2009) Ghrelin and apolipoprotein AIV levels show opposite trends to leptin levels during weight loss in morbidly obese patients. *Obes Surg* **19**(10): 1414–1423.

22. Gagné DJ, Papasavas PK, Dovec EA, Urbandt JE, Caushaj PF. (2009) Effect of immunosuppression on patients undergoing bariatric surgery. *Surg Obes Relat Dis* **5**(3): 339–345.

23. Rochester D, Jain A, Polotsky AJ *et al.* (2009) Partial recovery of luteal function after bariatric surgery in obese women. *Fertil Steril* **92**(4): 1410–1415.

24. Escobar-Morreale HF, Botella-Carretero JI, Alvarez-Blasco F, Sancho J, San Millán JL. (2005) The polycystic ovary syndrome associated with morbid obesity may resolve after weight loss induced by bariatric surgery. *J Clin Endocrinol Metab* **90**(12): 6364–6369.

25. Eid GM, Cottam DR, Velcu LM, Mattar SG, Korytkowski MT, Gosman G, Hindi P, Schauer PR. (2005) Effective treatment of polycystic ovarian syndrome with Roux-en-Y gastric bypass. *Surg Obes Relat Dis* **1**(2): 77–80.

26. Wilson-Pérez HE, Seeley RJ. (2011) The Effect of vertical sleeve gastrectomy on a rat model of polycystic ovarian syndrome. *Endocrinol* **152**(10): 3700–3705.

Index

A

adjustable gastric band, 69, 113, 140

B

Bariatric, 67–74
Bariatric Complications, 77–79, 81, 83–86, 88, 90, 93
bariatric diet, 114, 117
bariatric surgery, 40, 43, 97–99, 103, 107–109, 113–114, 121, 124–126, 130–132, 138, 141, 147–148, 151–153, 155–156
Biliopancreatic Diversion and Duodenal Switch, 37
BPD/DS, 38, 40–48, 51

D

diet related complications, 113
duodenal switch, 37–38

E

enteroinsulin axis, 38, 42, 44

G

gastric band, 78, 84
gastric bypass, 29, 68–70, 72–73
gastrojejunostomy, 29, 31–32
gastroplasty, 15–17, 19, 22

H

Historical procedures, 17, 19, 20–23

J

Jejunoileal Bypass, 12

L

Laparoscopic Bariatric Surgery, 50
leak, 78, 86–89, 93

M

macronutrients, 125
metabolic changes, 148, 151
micronutrients, 118–120

O

obesity, 68, 70–71, 73–74, 148,
    150–154
obesity-related health risks, 1

R

Randomized control trials (RCTs),
    67–68, 71–73
revision, 84, 90–91, 93
Roux-en-Y gastric bypass (RYGB),
    29, 78, 113

S

Sleeve gastrectomy, 55, 69, 72–73,
    113, 138
stricture, 89–91, 93
Super Morbid Obesity, 38

W

weight loss, 68, 70–71, 73
weight loss surgery diet, 113